FIVE EMPOWERING PRINCIPLES OF ACTION RESEARCH THAT LEAD TO SUCCESSFUL PERSONAL AND PROFESSIONAL DEVELOPMENT

Yoshihiko Ariizumi

University Press of America,® Inc.
Lanham · Boulder · New York · Toronto · Oxford

Copyright © 2005 by
University Press of America,® Inc.
4501 Forbes Boulevard
Suite 200
Lanham, Maryland 20706
UPA Acquisitions Department (301) 459-3366

PO Box 317
Oxford
OX2 9RU, UK

All rights reserved
Printed in the United States of America
British Library Cataloging in Publication Information Available

Library of Congress Control Number: 2005927672
ISBN: 978-0-7618-3233-1

∞™ The paper used in this publication meets the minimum
requirements of American National Standard for Information
Sciences—Permanence of Paper for Printed Library Materials,
ANSI Z39.48—1984

To my father

Whose influence I could not see much when he was around,
But now I feel it stronger when he is gone

Contents

Preface ix
Acknowledgements xi

Introduction 1
    Action Research as a Bridge 2
    The Illustration of Traditional Science 3
    Action Research as Creator of Knowledge 5
    Pitfalls of the Procedure-centered Approach 5
    Major Focus of This Book 7
    Chigen（知源）: A concept that represents
    a more holistic understanding of human behaviors 9

Chapter One: Ownership with Accountability 13
    Securing Ownership in Action Research 14
    Function of Ownership in Action Research 16
    Ways to Nurture Ownership 16
    Action Research as a Moral Science 19
    Growth of Chigen with Ownership with
    Accountability 20
    Questions & Activities for Better Understanding 22

Chapter Two: Mastering Locality and Context 23

Chapter Two: Mastering Locality and Context 23
    The Status of Local Knowledge 24
    Importance of Local Knowledge 24
    Learning at a Specific Locality 26
    Why Do General Laws Often Fail to Work at a Locality, While Action Research Addresses Local Issues Successfully? 27
    Questions & Activities for Better Understanding 30

Chapter Three: Total Engagement in Practice 33
    Characteristics of Practice 35
    Messiness 35
    Nonlinearity 36
    Dynamism 36
    Unpredictability 37
    Multi-dimensionality and the Total Involvement of the Self 39
    The Role of Feelings 41
    Tacit Knowledge 42
    Objectivity 43
    Subjectivity 44
    Free Agency 46
    Refined Subjectivity 47
    Morality and Spirituality 48
    Relevance 54
    The Relationship between Practice and Chigen 56
    Conclusions 57
    Questions & Activities for Better Understanding 59

Chapter Four: Growing Through Dialectic Process 61
    Questions & Activities for Better Understanding 69

Chapter Five: Systematic Reflection 71
    Summery 82
    Questions & Activities for Better Understanding 83

Chapter Six: Lived Experience of Action Research 85
    Tutoring 88
    Fatherhood 89
    Family Game 92

Facilitation of a Student's Implementation 94
  Professional Performance 96
  Questions & Activities for Better Understanding 98

Bibliography 101

Index 113

About the Author 117

Preface

You probably have some important matter(s) (relationships, careers, hobbies, etc.) in your life in which you care about the quality of your engagement and performance. The true sense of happiness and joy seems deeply rooted in the outcomes of these matters. When you feel constant and steady improvement in your dealings with these matters, you become hopeful and have a sense of fulfillment.

After decades of search for better ways to improve such matters in my life and in those of others, I finally came across action research, which looked enigmatic at that time, since I could not find any simple and clear definition among hundreds of professional writings on it. Yet, I was attracted deeply by this new improvement mode of matters because hundreds of testimonials by action researchers suggested to me that there was something tremendously powerful in action research.

During the next four years while I was enrolled in a doctorate program I conducted an epistemological study of action research. In other words, my main objective at that time was to find out what action research really is. This kind of investigation is never ending as philosophical questions like "What is time?" can be addressed in an infinite number of ways. Therefore, instead of attaining a single clear-cut definition, I ferreted out a diverse action research variety. Nonetheless, the end results were not as hopeless as I had expected them to be. Through analyzing hundreds of testimonials, I found out that I could extract major components that could make action research meaningful and productive. My ensuing case studies that are introduced in Chapter Six validate these components.

After writing the first draft of this manuscript, I started several new action research projects—some of which were personal and others collaborative—which are not contained in this book. I discovered, interestingly enough, that the projects were increasingly successful and empowering as I became more comfortable with the procedure. The process of revising this manuscript made me more conscious of these empowering principles, and with this new insight, I was able to more carefully apply these principles. The results were phenomenal. I witnessed that I was more naturally and comfortably employing action research, and that my collaborators were increasingly energized and committed in their endeavors.

As I will reiterate in the following comments, action research is not a quick remedy. Procedure-based applications tend to be inefficient. Only when we carefully apply those principles, will we be surprised by the repeated break-through that we will unexpectedly experience in the process of action research.

I believe that if we provide a good facilitator, even 5th or 6th graders can acquire basic skills to conduct meaningful action research. Perhaps, any adult practitioner can perform action research if they are appropriately trained. As many users once shared one computer (main frame), and later the personal computer became a norm, I hope that the same change will happen with action research. The day may come when action research is taught in public education as one of the literacy skills.

As far as I know, this book is the first attempt of this kind to invite readers to employ action research in the broadest and most flexible way in their personal and professional endeavors.

Acknowledgments

The foremost thanks must go to my mentor, Professor Dillon Inouye of Brigham Young University for his wonderful and enlightening guidance that has led me to numerous innovative ideas including action research, and I am also heavily indebted to him for further advice—including this book project. The next thanks goes to Professor Stefinee Pinnegar of Brigham Young University who not only served as my academic advisory committee member during my doctorate study but also gave me encouragement and advised me to continue my action research and publish my findings.

As English is my second language, it has been an enormous challenge to organize my ideas into expressions in a language that is foreign to me. I express my warmest gratitude for my editors: Mr. Arlie Capps, Mrs. Sue Varley, Mr. John LaMont, and Maria, my daughter.

It would have been impossible for this longitudinal project to have persisted so long without the positive feedback from my friends and associates. Among those friends, James Goodman and George Hudak were particularly noteworthy for their sincere interest and willingness to apply the principles of action research in their professional lives. I would also like to include all of my colleagues in the Foreign Languages and Literatures Department of Lafayette College who have shared with me many insightful suggestions and recommendations that have helped me improve the quality of my writing.

Special thanks to my students; they have been my collaborators, and some of them allowed me to facilitate their personal action research projects. These experiences have been invaluable in my study to validate the five principles of action research. I would like to name a few of them for the significance of their contribution to my experience: Sarah Nakanishi, Tana Zerr, Mary Taylor, Hiroyuki Kiyono, Victor Mrosso, Cathy Schubel, and Andrew McCarty.

Finally I would like to express my appreciation for my family. They have been positive and helpful throughout my engagement in various personal action-research projects. In addition to the aforementioned editing by Maria, my son, Joshua, offered technical support while I was preparing the original manuscript and my wife, Shizuko, has always propelled me to work faster and maintain focus. Without their constant efforts, the completion of this book would have been much longer in coming.

Introduction

Action Research—Widely Known, Yet Not Well Understood

There has been marked growth in the interest and application of action research during the last two decades. Is this another vogue that comes and goes away? Are there any elements in action research that can be carried into the new century to generate new perspectives, improve practice, and enrich life? Documents that apply action research are characterized by their meaning and relevance to their subject of study. Nonetheless, deeper understanding may be more elusive. Even after reading success stories and step-by-step guidelines, an observer may still wonder what makes action research efficacious. Recognition of its usefulness does not always correspond with an understanding of its nature. We often trust a thing because those whom we trust recommend it, or because it happened to work when we tried it. A pain reliever, for example, is believed to be useful as long as it functions as expected. We may not be concerned much with why and how it works when we are in pain. However, to use it more effectively requires some medical expertise, including the knowledge of why and how it works. The same is true with action research. A wise and creative use of action research must be based on deeper understanding of its essential characteristics. Unfortunately, action research may be widely recognized as a useful instrument to improve practice, but it has hardly been explored and explained in depth.

You may have learned about action research before. You may have experienced some aspects of it. Or you may have experienced improvements in your practice through aspects of action research without recognizing them as such. Whatever your experience, this new field called action research can promise improvements in your life. The uniqueness of action research is that the knower plays a significant part in the known. Two well-known authors defined action research as a deliberate, solution-oriented investigation that is group- or personally owned and conducted. It is characterized by spiraling cycles of problem identification, systematic data collection, reflection, analysis, data-driven action taken, and, finally, problem redefinition. The linking of the terms "action" and "research" highlights the essential features of this method: trying out ideas in practice as a means of increasing knowledge about and/or improving curriculum, teaching, and learning (Kemmis & McTaggart 1982). Thus the traditional conception of objectivity as a foundation of sciences is altered in the potential of action research to empower the individual.

Action Research as a Bridge

Action research can be conceived as a bridge over a chasm, connecting the seemingly unconnectable. On one side of the gorge there are ethereal or abstract concepts such as theory, generalizable ideas, objective knowledge, etc. The other side has many down-to-earth concrete concepts like specific action, particular practice, or day-to-day activity. Traditionally, these two realms have been completely separate. In academia people abstract general rules from reality and disseminate them to the world. On the other side practitioners tackle moment-to-moment problems to achieve locally defined objectives. The chief concern of the practitioner is to successfully implement ideas to manage the local reality. With abstracting on one side and practical, real-world application on the other, the boundary between these two realms has always been clearly demarcated. Consequently, changing roles from one realm to the other is somewhat difficult, and is rarely achieved. Such a distinction has become stronger over the last few millennia. As specialization has increasingly become the norm in society, this gap has only become wider. Academia has become more dominant in the creation of new knowledge, and its esoteric language has often marginalized the practitioners, who have become consumers rather than producers of new knowledge. Thus the gorge has become wider and deeper, a barrier to innovation in a local practice. How can action research bridge such a prodigious gap?

This book invites readers to understand action research in forms usually hidden from casual observation. Only since late in the last century has objective knowledge ceased to dominate, and the idea of neutral or objective observation, despite of different standpoints, has been severely scrutinized and refuted both in the social sciences and in the physical sciences. Although the natural sciences have successfully innovated our understanding of our physical surroundings and even succeeded in reaching the moon, social sciences focus on human beings who can choose to act for or against the natural laws. General theories fail to predict individual behaviors at specific situations. Action research can form a basis for such prediction.

The illusion of Traditional Scientific Approach

Illusion occurs when we cross over an unexamined boundary. A toddler may mimic a comic hero by attempting to fly, crossing the boundary of his physical strength and the law of gravity, and thus falling to the ground. Almost a century ago, many people who attempted to fly were injured or killed until they finally employed technology to enable them to fly. Human history has innumerable examples of those who crossed boundaries with tragic results. Some acted out of mere folly, but there were pioneers who lost their lives in heroic struggles and left a legacy of knowledge that marked the boundaries they crossed. However noble their action in crossing a boundary, illusion is still illusion. If a boundary is already known, we should search for it to avoid the danger and waste. In this book, readers will find the way to identify what the boundary is when they apply so-called "scientific knowledge" to their specific problems. If they then perform action research in their practice, it will illuminate the boundary.

There are countless boundaries in our lives. We cross the boundary when we buy clothes simply because they are in fashion or because we think people wearing them look attractive. We cross the boundary when we work longer, neglecting our family, simply because we see everybody around is working longer. We cross the boundary when we start an e-business simply because doing so is fashionable. In summary, we cross the boundary when we employ some idea in our particular situation simply because we witnessed that it worked for another person in a particular situation. Is it a bad thing to try someone else's ideas or to follow someone else's example? Absolutely not—if it is considered in itself. This human tendency to imitate others can be a great asset for personal growth as long as it is properly controlled. One of the positive facets of this human characteristic is called "self-efficacy," (a self-belief of one's capability to perform a specific task) a concept that deeply engaged a leading social psychologist, Albert Bandura. He observed how self-efficacy is enhanced through mutual influence among peers. Certainly this human tendency has great potential that we can utilize to grow, while still remaining within the boundaries. Doesn't general knowledge of sciences inform us about those boundaries so that we can have better control?

Yes, the sciences provide a plethora of information, including information pertaining to the boundaries relevant to our unique situation. However, very often, available knowledge does not serve well in our particular circumstances. Let me illustrate this by my own predicament. I am of average height for a Japanese man of my age. My arm is only a little shorter in proportion to my height than arms of most Japanese men, but exceptionally short compared to typical American proportions. I may visit a dozen local clothing stores, but I never find a regular ready-made shirt that fits me. Nevertheless, I have to buy American shirts to replace my old Japanese shirts. To avoid extra expense, I have two options. One is to beg my wife to do the alteration, and the other is to put up with uncomely and inconvenient sleeves sticking out from under my Japanese suit. Living in a foreign country, this is a recurring nuisance for me. For most of American readers, it may not be a problem at all to find clothes to fit. But it may be more difficult to find a good "fit" for your specific practice among hundreds of thousands of ideas that are created every year. Usually these ideas are generated as ready-made knowledge for general purposes. They seldom address local issues. They may be accompanied with suggestions for different applications. However, their categorization is rough at best. Tailoring is the consumers' responsibility. Scientific or general knowledge may present us knowledge about boundaries, but they are usually very rough estimates, often too rough for our immediate use. How can we tailor such knowledge?

Action Research as Creator of Knowledge

There are two different ways to approach this problem. One is to adjust a ready-made idea for local needs through a standard alteration, as my wife does with my shirtsleeves, which fixes only salient problems. This approach is similar to that of the applied sciences, which provide a standardized rough fit. The other is to obtain order-made knowledge based on the local needs. This sounds expensive, but you can imagine how comfortable you would feel in that knowledge. This is the expediency of action research. Action research creates and tailors knowledge according to local needs.

This book gives you fresh insight into areas where action research can make significant differences in your practice. It also guides you to essential components and potentials of action research that make it a unique and powerful tool. This book describes and expands those principles of action research on which you can base your own most meaningful improvement projects. Although the purpose of this book is not to provide step-by-step procedures to conduct action research, you can find useful information about related resources in the bibliography.

Pitfalls of the Procedure-centered Approach

Before further discussions, a few cautions are in order. People may easily develop misconceptions about action research when they focus only on the procedure and ignore the principles behind it. It is true that step-by-step procedures are easy to understand and follow. However, there are dangers and limitations in procedure-centered approaches. Mechanical, rigid adherence to the guidelines sacrifices the holistic understanding, loses sight of the priority, and puts unnecessary constraints on our practice. For example, the following diagram (Figure 1) based on the ideas created by Kurt Lewin (1890-1947), represents the process accurately yet contains a pitfall that traps those whose understanding is superficial.

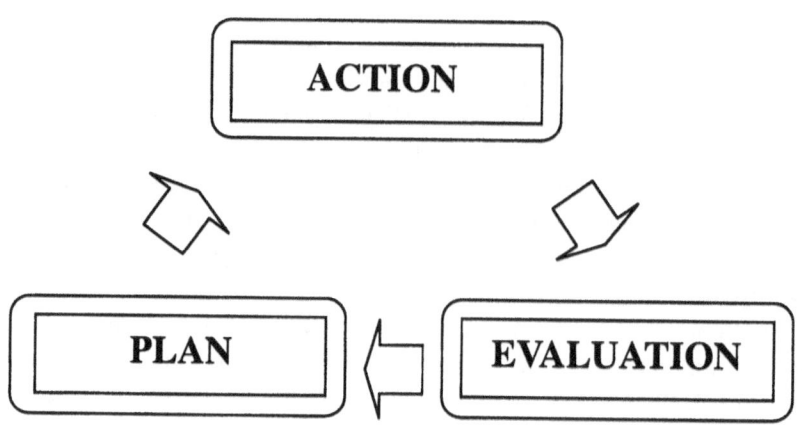

Figure 1

For example, Ken, a teacher, applies action research in his practice by following the diagram. He implements a so-called teacher-proof system in his classroom. Ken slavishly follows the prescribed plan. He also prepares a rigid evaluative procedure to compare the outcomes with those of the traditional approach, hoping to obtain scientifically valid information about his new experience. Actions are taken according to the plan, and the results are analyzed carefully and reported to an external audience. Can this process still be called action research? It is true that there are dozens of different types of action research, and many people define action research quite differently. Nevertheless, there are three fundamental flaws in concluding that Ken conducted meaningful action research. First, action research gains its power through repetition of the process. Without going through a few cycles, a significant effect may not be observed; action research is a process of refinement. Second, at this stage the local knowledge generated by the action research has not played a significant role in decision-making and action. Finally, Ken's way of implementing the results of his action research, at least at this stage, may not serve well for the local reality. The direct implementation of someone else's idea, the rigidity of the evaluative method, and the demand of reporting to the external audience may put an unreasonably heavy burden on Ken while he is probably struggling with his demanding teaching responsibilities.

Here is the danger. By following the prescribed procedure, you may be forced to unreasonably stretch your effort to fit the prescription. Additionally, by being overly concerned with the external audience, you may neglect the internal needs in your practice. If you employ a principle-based approach, however, you have more freedom to choose. You can customize your action research according to specific, local circumstances.

With that said, one should be careful not go too far. Do not give up the idea to try action research in your practice prematurely because of the demanding conditions of your practice. Who is too busy to sharpen his/her tools when they have become too dull to function effectively? We should always make time to improve our practice, because such an investment, we know, will be profitable over time. I have a strong conviction that action research is a wise investment applicable everywhere in the personal and social life of those who consider their practice to be important.

Action research is not a panacea. Action research can provide excellent opportunities only where we can efficiently and thoroughly investigate not only the target of the action, but also the practitioners themselves. In order to accomplish the most desirable outcomes, action research must be based on the pro-active stance of the practitioner. Action research provides many avenues for investigation beyond cognitive perspectives, including emotions, value systems, and most essential matters of our existence. Since action research directs time and effort from other activities, we must think carefully about balancing action research with other aspects of our lives.

The Major Focus of This Book

This book is based on an attempt to restore personhood to the role of practitioner/researcher in order to support the validity of using personal knowledge to improve practice. Action research always involves human beings, and practice improves more or less according to human changes, which presuppose changes in personal knowledge and perspective. Action research does not always look for objective, detached knowledge; it often focuses on helping personal knowledge to grow. It is a mode of action in which we see reality through more refined lenses.

After careful examination of hundreds of articles and continuous refinement of each concept, I have extracted five essential principles that make action research effective and meaningful:

1. Ownership with Accountability
2. Mastering Locality and Context

3. Total Engagement in Practice
4. Growing through Dialectical Process
5. Systematic Reflection

Action research should start with ownership of the research. Without ownership deep learning is not likely to occur, and such learning is the basis of improvement and growth. However, there should be some qualifications with regard to this ownership; irresponsible ownership is not ownership at all. Accountability is complementary to ownership in this first component. Locality clearly distinguishes action research from traditional positivistic research, which has been the foundation of technological development for a long time. Locality and context interact in endless complexity, creating an infinite source of learning. Total engagement in practice contributes more to the unique quality of action research than any other component. The knowledge that comes through practice is often mysterious, being full of tacit elements. The unarticulated may be the more abundant part of this knowledge. The total involvement of a person, where the person must be seen more holistically than is traditional, characterizes this component. Dialectical process is always present to some degree in experiential learning. Action research, however, conscientiously utilizes this mechanism of development. Terms such as *cycle*, *spiral*, *reflexivity*, and *dialogue* are often used to denote this mechanism. The last component, systematic reflection typically distinguishes action research from general experiential learning. It also lifts the resultant knowledge to a higher level of validity both to the practitioners themselves and to others. Reflection can take place at any stage of the research, but it should be systematically built into the process. It becomes most meaningful when it happens in three different modes: record, review, and report.

Action research and ordinary experiential learning have a great deal in common. The difference is seemingly minute, yet its significance is enormous. Action research requires extra data collection in a locally defined systematic way, yet this small methodological difference generates significant knowledge.

In this introductory chapter, the characteristics of action research have been outlined and their value has been discussed. It will be useful to introduce a new concept to express the goal of action research. When we decide whether or not action research is working in practice, we usually look at the resulting changes to the practice. It is generally more difficult to measure how much practitioners themselves have changed. However, the change in the practitioner is often a more reliable sign of a long-term improvement since the change in practice depends on innumerable situational factors that are constantly in a state of flux. Moreover, if we can focus on the personal traits that directly lead to intelligent judgments and performances, we can more accurately assess how well action research is functioning. How do we designate this set of human traits? Since there is no word in English that exactly represents such a construct, I believe it is appropriate to introduce some foreign terminology.

Chigen（知源）: A Concept That Represents a More Holistic Understanding of Human Behaviors

立会いに臨んでは、見の目を弱く、観の目を強く持つべし。
Tachiai ni nozonde wa ken no me o yowaku, kan no me o tsuyoku motsu beshi.
(In a fight, view the opponent more holistically rather than analytically. Miyamoto Musashi, 1584-1645)

Musashi, arguably the strongest sword fighter in the history of Japanese warriors, who is also known for his painting and writing, revealed in the statement above one of his techniques summarized in his final book, called *The Book of Five Rings*. In any practice, when we lose the holistic view and become preoccupied in details of an event, we increase our likelihood of failure. To engage in a practice is to be involved in multiple concepts. Not only does the practitioner have unique personal traits, but also each event includes an infinite number of factors, uniquely arranged and correlated; any single formula or strategy cannot lead us successfully through an event of practice. Many attempts have been made in the past to identify important personal traits, knowledge, and skills for excellent practice. However, none of these attempts has produced a comprehensive list that covers all aspects of performance. Nor can these attempts collectively do so. No theory can perfectly explain the phenomena of practice.

In perceiving practice as a phenomenon, I began to wonder if there is a better way to look at the entire situation behind successful practice. I decided I would do better to designate the entirety without identifying the individual elements that comprise it. I named it *Chigen*（知源）using two Chinese characters. *Chi*（知）represents *intelligence*（英知）and *gen*（源）means *source*. *Chigen* is a construct that is supposed to exist in us and enables any intelligent or purposeful action. I intend to use this concept as a 'black box' (in which its function is known but its inner working can not be seen) through which any intelligent or meaningful action can emerge. Although many theorists imply some entity that "creates and recreates schemes," "theorizes phenomena," or "judges various options to choose the best to handle a situation," their focus is on functions. Usually they do not identify what is behind such functions, and these functions significantly lean to the cognitive. Heidegger's *Dasein* is similar to

Chigen in scope and comprehensiveness, but Chigen focuses specifically on the entity of the being behind any intelligent behavior that leads practice to success.

Examples may help us understand the kinds of concepts represented by Chigen. For instance, we can learn to ride a bicycle, but we cannot explain verbally everything that someone else needs to know to learn to ride a bicycle. Knowledge that cannot be communicated verbally is called *tacit knowledge* (See Polanyi 1958). Tacit knowledge does not belong exclusively to the cognitive domain, yet it does belong to Chigen. Is tacit knowledge equivalent to skill, then? No. In the example of bicycle riding, while tacit knowledge is part of the skill, the skill also includes good coordination, clear eyesight, and so forth. Then does this skill belong to Chigen? The answer is yes.

Suppose a little girl is attempting to train a dog. Because she is impatient, she fails to teach the dog the trick she would like. Then her father tries the same thing, and because of his maturity in controlling his emotions and training patiently, he succeeds. His patience enables him to lead the dog to the point where it can master the trick. The father's patience embodies both emotional and spiritual traits, which also belong to Chigen.

The next example may help to illustrate the breadth of this concept. Our outdoor cat has learned that she can effectively wake us during the night if she climbs up to the bedroom windows to meow when she finds no food. We are not sure how much of her behavior can be explained by instinct, but obviously she has learned our behavior so that she knows where we usually are at night. Without excluding the instinct aspect of her behavior, we can say that Chigen is at work in this case. Chigen does not differentiate instinctive from learned behaviors as they lead to intelligent and wise behaviors. We define Chigen in such a way that whatever leads to such a behavior, even to a smallest degree, is included in it. Also we cannot separate instinct from reason in Chigen because they are sometimes interactive. When a mother is caring for her child, for instance, we do not have to separate the maternal instinctive aspect of her behavior from the reasoning aspect.

Traditional scientific approaches to innovation are to impose external or general ideas on practice to produce improvements. In contrast, action research mainly employs internal or local ideas of the practitioners in improving their practice. Thus action research enriches and refines a practitioner's Chigen along with technical changes in a practice situation so that practice moves to a higher level.

The key to success in dealing with human behavior is to maintain a holistic view like Musashi's Kan, which led him to repeated victory. Instead of seeing different elements of our behavior separately, we need to see them in a vision of wholeness. This does not mean that we should neglect analysis of details. Any practitioner in any field may find that an intensive drill in one segment of behavior or an extensive study of one content area can greatly enhance overall performance in practice. However, it is apparent that drill and specific knowledge do not solve all the problems of practice. Additionally, they do not help the practitioner sequence and prioritize actions. But if we look at the practitioner's Chigen in its entirety, we find endless options to improve from which we may choose the most appropriate, effective, and efficient approach. Ownership helps us tap such a reservoir of opportunities to grow. As long as we keep track of the development of Chigen, we are likely to see gradual yet continuous and natural improvement of practice.

The following five chapters will view action research through the windows of five principles and describe how action research helps Chigen grow.

Chapter One

Ownership with Accountability

An activity cannot be classified as meaningful action research without ownership. True ownership accompanied by accountability ensures meaningful learning that leads to fundamental improvements in practice. The history of the world is filled with countless examples that affirm the importance of ownership for human development. Toward the end of the last century, we witnessed the corruption and collapse of communist systems in which people lacked true ownership/accountability. We learned that such systems eventually fail to maintain high human performance not only in productivity but also in other qualities.

Failures due to the lack of ownership are not limited to communist, socialist, totalitarian or militaristic societies. For example, in Japan miraculous changes were brought about by the privatization of the railway system. The new system allowed more authentic ownership/accountability for the workers and leaders alike when the government decided to sell the national railway system to the private sector. Previously, Japan had incurred huge deficits through the national railway operation. The shift of ownership was immediately followed by tremendous changes. The system was streamlined. Many creative ideas were implemented. Within a few years the system was completely transformed into profitable cooperative structures with much better services. Large organizations are not the only examples. We daily encounter many episodes and incidents that show that ownership brings excitement, commitment, and true growth to our children and to others.

Securing Ownership in Action Research

Existence of ownership is shown by the degree of agency or freedom that a practitioner may have in the action research. When a practitioner has ownership, he/she can learn about the action research, use it, and change it at will. One expert defined ownership for practitioners in action research as the right to select their focus and decide their agenda (Noffke, 1995). For example, if someone forces you against your will to perform research-based improvement in your practice, your ownership is seriously diminished. If factors other than the demands of your practice continuously interfere with the action research procedure, your ownership is in danger. From the facilitator's point of view, if your practitioners are passively or reluctantly responding to your suggestions to implement action research, even if they appear to be following an action research procedure, they are not experiencing true ownership. Even a positive and willing attitude may not guarantee true ownership if they are not accompanied by the skills and understanding necessary to conduct action research properly and independently.

Let us go back to a fundamental question to ensure more careful, targeted discussion. What does it mean to "own" action research? Ownership in action research mainly means two things: the ownership of practice procedures and the ownership of research procedures. Action researchers must have control over their practice. Reaching this goal involves overcoming a number of obstacles. Since our practice exists within multiple organizations, e.g., the work place, the community, a city, a state, a nation, and so forth—each level constricts us in one way or another with its rules and regulations. In addition, our action research partners or supervisors may also bring requests (some may be unreasonable and peculiar) into our practice. Thus perfect control over the entire practice is a dream. Nonetheless, our chance to gain some control is a significant one. Adapting a positive proactive stance with enthusiasm opens up countless opportunities for control.

In fact, external constrains do not hamper the ownership of action research as seriously as internal discordance. Suppose we are in jail. That means we are in one of the worst conditions to exercise control in our practice, which may be simply to perform what is required for a prisoner. Can we apply action research to this practice? There is a myriad of ways to conduct action research even in such confinement. Establishing communication, maintaining physical and mental health, dealing with solitude, and being productive with the 'free' time of imprisonment may be among those areas to study and improve. The prisoner can create as many sub-categories to study as he or she likes. History teaches us how to be a productive inmate. Joseph who was sold to Egypt as recorded in Genesis, Indian Prime Minister Nehru (1889-1964), and Emmanuel Levinas (1905-1995) are just a few among many whose imprisonment was used productively to prepare them for their successful future. In contrast, internal factors can be more detrimental. Feigned motivation and deficient rationale can produce nothing but a waste of valuable time and efforts.

The other form of ownership involves the research process. Owning the research refers to the right to choose the problems for study, the method for collecting data, the way of interpreting the research results, and the way of applying the findings. But such ownership also assumes responsibility for the research effects. Once you gain control over even a small portion of a practice, you can find innumerable ways of framing research in that given segment. Again, it is not external conditions of the practitioner that limit the research potentials; it is his/her internal barriers such as mental block or lack of imagination and skills in conducting action research.

As the previous discussions have implied, it is not always easy to secure true ownership of either sort, even harder when they are combined into action research. False ownership easily slips into practice while we are tackling day-to-day problems. Therefore from time to time practitioners must carefully examine their motives for engaging in action research. Motivation must be intrinsic, arising from the practitioner's immediate needs, concerns, and interests. The challenge for facilitators is even greater, since it requires moral strength not to exploit their practitioners. Facilitators must constantly monitor the locus of ownership so as not to intrude into the practitioners' right to do their own action research. Successful maintenance of ownership demands empathy from facilitators.

Function of Ownership in Action Research

Why is ownership so important? It is obvious that without ownership what we learn from action research may be, at best, partial and superficial. If ownership is to help our learning reach completion and depth, what is the process? The next example illustrates this point. When we travel to a new destination by car as a passenger, often we do not remember the route well. However, when we drive ourselves, our memory of the route is much more complete. As a passenger we do not own the process of driving, nor do we feel much accountability for arriving at the destination. Owning the driving makes us more alert and attentive to traffic, signs, landmarks, and other details of the route. With ownership the consequences of our actions belong to us: Ownership brings with it accountability. If we take a wrong turn, we may get lost and waste time and energy, which may cause distress and frustration. This potential negative consequence fuels our alertness and attentiveness to our driving. Thus ownership leads to more authentic learning, which is a basis of action research. Any practitioner who has ownership feels more strongly bound to his or her practice, developing stronger intent, commitment, and motivation.

In summary, ownership helps to generate knowledge that is more accurate, focused, coherent, and integrated, as well as deeper and more complete. It engenders confidence, autonomy and initiative, and it deeply affects the emotions of practitioners so that the change hits the very core of their existence.

Ways to Nurture Ownership

Even though ownership is so essential to meaningful action research, it is not automatic, even when it is offered. It is not easy to promote ownership, especially when action research is initiated externally. Some people are reluctant to increase ownership, increasing responsibility and problems as well. Too much ownership at the beginning of a new project can overwhelm and discourage novice action researchers. On the other hand, facilitators can exploit practitioners by not giving them enough ownership. Therefore, an action research facilitator needs to use careful thought in dealing with people, continually monitoring the locus of ownership. Wells (1994) suggests, "The principle criterion for evaluating a piece of action research is not the significance of its finding for others, but rather the value of the experience of undertaking it for the researcher him/herself" (p. 28).

Is there any way for us to keep track of the locus of ownership? Is there any sign that will reveal true ownership? When we search for essential signs of ownership in the action research process, we notice that there is a function that can hardly be imitated by a false ownership. I will call this function "focalization/problematization." "Focalization" is a mental function that selects a certain issue about our practice as a focal point for research. We usually focus on one thing at a time. That focus shows our interest. So the first step is to ask a practitioner to describe the point(s) of interest in his/her research. The second step is to check whether that described interest really matches the action. This step is necessary for the two major reasons. First, practitioners often do not know what their real interest is, and their interest may change over the time. Second, there is often a political dimension to the relationship between facilitators and practitioners. Practitioners, as subordinates, may find it difficult to express their real concern when they think that such a remark might offend their supervisors.

"Problematization" is similar to focalization. This function uniquely frames the focal issue(s). The same issue can be addressed through problematization in a variety of ways while focalization is simply to turn attention to the issue. You can approach it positively or negatively. Your attitude, value judgment, and preference make your problematization unique. In a sense your self is revealed in the way you problematize the issue. The same two-step process can check whether or not the problematization reflects true ownership. You can ask a practitioner how he/she addresses the focal issue, then follow up to verify the point.

It is likely that FP (Focalization/Problematization) will shift from one point to another multiple times as action research advances. Such shifts are necessary for action research to improve practice by assisting practitioners' personal and professional development. Therefore, the attitude of both facilitators and practitioners should be open and positive. A flexible research agenda is desirable. Facilitators are responsible for creating a climate that encourages free expression of ideas and feelings. FP points are defined and redefined progressively. Action research adds any different dimensions to a practice including that of self-examination.

Only the person with true ownership can have ideal freedom to pursue for a high-leveraged solution while he or she is identifying an FP point. Ownership provides an opportunity to be proactive. There is usually no external compulsion to improve in an area of practice that action research may identify. The improvement that action research aims at is a matter of choice for that action researcher. He or she can conduct the action research without worry, because no one else is concerned with the outcomes as long as he or she does not adversely affect the practice. The sense of failure is less likely to be experienced as long as the action researcher does not have unreasonable expectations for his or her endeavor. Ownership protects action researchers from the intrusion by others. Constructive criticism may be welcomed from others, which is far more beneficial than self-contentment. However, until you are ready to face more severe challenges, you can maintain your experience with a positive tone of satisfaction, enjoyment, and excitement. You have control over the situation because of the ownership.

Action research accompanied by true ownership creates a defensive mechanism as well as an intriguing environment conducive to testing new ideas. Two contrasting situations will illustrate how action research can serve as a buffer against criticisms. Situation One: You receive a blow to your stomach unexpectedly. Situation Two: You are prepared for a blow with hardened abdominal muscles. There is a difference between these two situations in the damage that the blow can cause. Action research with appropriate ownership prepares practitioners for criticism. Through action research, a frame of mind is developed in which criticisms are constructively accepted. Action research raises the practitioners' awareness of the local phenomena of practice, including their strengths and weaknesses, and this awareness leads them to deeper understanding of themselves. Such an understanding guards them against potentially damaging criticisms. In an ordinary practice mode, while practitioners' attentions are totally consumed in their demanding day-to-day tasks, even constructive criticisms often result in no positive effects. In contrast, serious action research often leads practitioners to deep self-reflection, highlighting their problems and initiating a search for solutions. Without this process a criticism is more likely to be disregarded, and the opportunity for improvement will be lost. Ownership creates a space with freedom and security: freedom to explore and examine local reality; freedom to reflect on performance individually; security of not being subjected to others' research agenda.

Where there is genuine ownership, there is perfect freedom of choice. Generally, training programs and workshops are, to a certain extent, imposed upon practitioners. In contrast, action research of one's own choice is perfectly flexible and can be customized to one's unique situation. There is no limit in such a choice about where to start action research. However, this does not preclude consulting with someone in deciding on a focus. Such consultation is perfectly appropriate.

Action Research as a Moral Science

This topic will be more fully discussed in Chapter Three; but it is appropriate to note here some issues that affect not only action researchers but also their facilitators since they both desire to continuously maintain optimal ownership. It is only right that ownership be accompanied by accountability, especially when we expect that an activity may cause significant personal or social consequences. Additionally, without mutual accountability we may not be able to maintain our ownership in a community. Thus ownership is intricately tied to moral issues.

True growth of a practitioner is only possible in the presence of ownership. To grant practitioners ownership is one of the best ways to honor their agency and to lead them to total involvement. Ownership motivates a strong commitment without which improvement may remain superficial.

Action research produces a subjective, value-laden view. And such a view often leads to the gain of personal and particular knowledge, based on which we make important decisions that change the course of our practice. It may sound contradictory, but the knowledge involved in action research is as biased and skewed as it is unique and distinctive (Reason 1993, 1262). While the traditional sciences carefully avoid "bias" and "skew," the human sciences such as action research have a much more positive aspect on these concepts. It is not that a human scientist embraces these two concepts that are generally conceived in a negative way. A human scientist will rather accept them as an inseparable part of human frailty while he or she is trying to overcome its weaknesses as much as possible. Apparently, it is not a neutral and universal idea but a bias-prone personal interpretation that actually affects or promotes the performance in a practice, which action research aims to enhance. Thus, we shift our reliance from method, which is neutral and universal, as the basis of knowing, to the human beings and the human community, which are always biased or skewed one way or another (Reason, 1993, 1259). Therefore, instead of discarding or neglecting biases and skews, action research tries to nurture an action researcher's biased and skewed view so that it becomes increasingly reasonable, realistic, and productive.

Another keyword—intention—will further clarify this subjectivity issue. Intention, which comes from the core of personhood, defines a focal point where action research generates new knowledge to improve the practice. Intention cannot be universal because it is not only restricted by its locality but also bound by its infallible attachment to the particular individual being. Intention cannot be neutral because the individual, from whom the intention is derived, has particular needs and desires that are constantly framing it.

Thus, when action researchers are granted ownership or they proactively gain it, more power is given to those fallible hands that control data management, decision-making, and implementation of new knowledge. Apparently, they assume more accountability and ethical responsibility while their improved practice affects others as well as themselves. As ownership gives more freedom for the agency to control and restricts the external intervention, action researchers have greater freedom to exercise their agency either for good or bad long-term consequences. Since the external regulations are minimized in the domain of an ownership-granted action research, there must be an alternative internal regulatory mechanism—ethical or moral strength—that keeps the endeavor from falling into chaos.

To conclude this section, let us summarize the major points. Inclusion of subjectivity or subjective judgments in the data collection, interpretation, and other processes distinguishes action research from traditional scientific approaches. Subjectivity is more meaningful and appropriate in action research because any given agent is an expert on his or her own perceptions and feelings while he or she is engaged in an action research, and those perceptions and feelings have a decisive role in the improvement of a practice. However, subjectivity has no meaning in the absence of freedom. Moreover, action researchers are free only when they are given or assume ownership. In fact, we cannot make practitioners acting agents without providing them ownership. Ownership is neither "free" nor easy to secure. Accountability is the price to obtain and maintain ownership. Securing the ownership for action researchers requires from the facilitators much moral strength, and likewise, accountability demands the same strength from the action researchers.

Growth of Chigen with Ownership and Accountability

When we are granted with ownership in action research, our Chigen will be more fully and deeply enriched. All of our faculties including feelings and physical abilities are more strongly involved. Let us take a close look at this growth process of Chigen. There is no doubt that the most authentic learning occurs at FP points. Those points, which can be anywhere in the practitioner's world, most actively engage the mind, and thus the most meaningful enrichment and growth of Chigen should happen around those points. However, these points are not necessarily part of the practice. Only ownership in action research can maintain those FP points within or in the vicinity of the practice. Therefore, ownership is one of the most critical enabling factors for the growth of Chigen, affecting Chigen in multiple ways. It affects not only human minds but also their emotions and spirits. It affects the entire existence of a practitioner. In sum, it affects Chigen holistically. To grant practitioners ownership is to provide their Chigen with the maximum opportunity to grow.

Questions & Activities for Better Understanding

> The following questions and suggestions are intended to stimulate further thinking. It may not be productive to follow them in a rigid manner. The readers are encouraged to modify questions/suggestions or create new questions/suggestions so that they can engage in truly meaningful thinking and learning.

1. Why is ownership so important for an action research to be successful? What kinds of benefit can we expect from obtaining and granting ownership in an action research?

2. In what situations is it problematic to maintain ownership? How can we overcome such difficult situations? Identify external and internal factors that prevent genuine ownership.

3. What are appropriate ways to look at biases and skews when we conduct an action research? Can we completely remove the influences of biases and skews? If not, how should we treat them?

4. If we, as facilitators, grant action researchers ownership without accountability, what might the consequences be? If we, as action researchers, take advantage of ownership but fail to be accountable, what kind of consequences must we face? What kind of moral strength should we have in order to secure and maintain ownership?

5. Why does monitoring the FP points help us ensure true ownership? Brainstorming sessions can provide excellent means to do this critical observation. What aspect of brainstorming can serve this purpose? What topics may be suitable for such a brainstorming session?

Chapter Two

Mastering Locality and Context

Once ownership is secured, the next step is to look at the immediate surroundings of practitioners to find where most meaningful action research can begin. Generally, people are not aware of the innumerable ways to tap the local reality of their practice so that they may obtain the most useful information to improve it. Most people fail in this respect simply because they do not know how to tap this rich source. In order to benefit more fully from their local experience, they must learn new skills, since such skills do not develop naturally. However inexhaustible the local knowledge base may be, it does not follow that general knowledge can be ignored, where "general" means that such knowledge is acquired from a publicly shared, well-examined, objective knowledge base. On the contrary, it is always desirable for local knowledge to be supported or complemented by general knowledge, otherwise practitioners' knowledge is inclined to be partial, myopic or biased. Therefore, in ideal action research, practitioners should know effective ways to learn from their local experience, maintaining a balance in using those two complementary knowledge sources. This challenging goal is only attainable when the researcher understands the mechanism through which local knowledge is produced and the way it can be complemented by general knowledge. Such understanding is the aim of this chapter.

The Status of Local Knowledge

Generally, local knowledge does not receive appropriate recognition in our society. Many consider local knowledge to be more naïve, easier to understand, or less important than esoteric knowledge. School education does not give sufficient emphasis to the value and utility of local knowledge. Children may be taught local history, or perform an occasional science experiment to retest the validity of a general theory at a local reality, or take a field trip to a nearby point of interest, but often they do not realize that these activities constitute vital learning. What is close to them seems elementary and plebeian. Classroom discussion, "show and tell,' and other performances that encourage individual knowledge and perceptions are conceived as pleasant indulgences or as stepping stones to "real" knowledge, rather than as chances to experience the value of local and first-hand knowledge. Individual students' remarks and questions and even teachers' accounts of their personal experiences never seem to gain a similar status to general knowledge, a fact evidenced by the lack of a formal testing procedure to examine such local knowledge. If one student shares his or her personal knowledge gained through experience, how do his or her classmates perceive such local knowledge? They decide personally whether or not they use such knowledge, but it usually does not find any official and legitimate place in the school curriculum.

In the context of action research, however, local or particular knowledge is highly valued, and general knowledge is often considered subsidiary: supporting local knowledge in solving local problems or validating the interpretation of local reality. All the knowledge available, first-hand and vicarious, local and general, may bear on a situation within a specific local context, but personal knowledge is the touchstone that guides the whole interpretive process.

Importance of Local Knowledge

The most effective improvements in practice are impossible without appropriate regard to local knowledge—the knowledge concerning a locality, the knowledge generated at a locality, a perspective from a locality, and so forth. Whatever innovative ideas we may develop based on the newest scientific findings, the application process will clash whenever local knowledge does not match in quality with these general ideas. Like the Biblical metaphor of "putting new wine into old bottles," mismatching the two constituent elements ruins the whole. Therefore, before utilizing general knowledge, we must enrich local knowledge in order to successfully interpret general knowledge into a local reality.

We should not underestimate local knowledge because it serves as an essential link between any useful idea (or any meaningful piece of general knowledge) and the local reality to which we are trying to implement such an idea or knowledge piece. Another reason to value local knowledge is the fact that the world is empty without local points. Analogously, the knowledge universe is constantly fed and examined by local knowledge, and without the latter, the former cannot exist without losing its validity.

The influence of local knowledge may go far beyond its local vicinity. Any location can be the source of ripples that affect the rest of the world. According to the Chaos Theory, a flip of a butterfly in Tokyo might cause a storm in New York City later. Consequences of each small incident at a locality and its knowledge can be far greater than we can imagine. Tradition and history are full of examples of the potential effects caused by groups of people, even of individuals, in remote localities. For example, Abraham from the Old Testament alone, in the midst of an unbelieving people, kept faithful and became the revered father of many nations, and the entire human family has been blessed by his legacy either directly or indirectly. Anne Sullivan taught the deaf-blind Helen Keller in a little corner of the world, but her efforts have given hope to countless people with severe handicaps worldwide. In the field of education we often underestimate the importance and richness of what is close to us.

The local point is uniquely connected with the rest of the world or universe. An infinite number of things can be learned from a single event in a locality; as Fleischer observed, "There may, indeed, be unlimited ways to 'read' our classroom research" (1995, 237). Of course, such an observation should not be limited to educational research. The same is true for any phenomenon of any practice. In any local context, original information, though inseparably connected with the world surrounding it, is still in its original and holistic state, rather than compartmentalized or decontextualized. This intact local reality provides a rich resource for study. We can examine this phenomenon from a different perspective. While the locality is exerting its influence on the surrounding world, the world is synchronously affecting it. This mutual relationship is endlessly complex. The context of any locality is unique, rich, and complex. Another educational example illustrates this point. "In their acts of being teacher, they are immersed," says Noffke, "in the totality of their educational situation, which is made up of all the elements that constitute their context, plus the past and possible future actions of other people" (1995, 134).

Learning at a Specific Locality

A specific locality is inexhaustibly describable. Once we start studying the phenomena associated with a locality, we can learn endlessly from it. We could begin a study from the perspective of any field: from mathematics through physics, biology, engineering, education, history, anthropology, sociology, economics, political science and so on. Each field has endless ramifications, and any locality can provide innumerable sources for the application of any field of study. The complex world of experiences must be valued; otherwise researchers may oversimplify the situation and prescribe incorrect approaches.   Knowledge is born at locality, like travelers' knowledge of an object of interest. Let us suppose that we are interested in an ancient mound in a great plain. We are approaching it in a car. At first, it is completely out of sight, but then from a certain distance we start seeing it. First, we see it vaguely as a dot. As we move closer, more details add to our perception. Later, we may spot a particular part of the mound. Then we shift our focus from one part to another. We may walk around on the mount measuring major objects. Eventually we may want to know the microscopic features of the soil and living organisms on the mound.

Knowledge develops at locality in two ways. The location functions as a background of the event and influences the knowledge that we obtain from the event. Then the knowledge is recast in a new, more densely textured form when we use it in practice (Brown, Collins, & Duguid, 1989, 33). Thus knowledge is created and refined in this two-way interaction between knowledge and the reality of practice. This process of refinement and creation can continue endlessly. Yet this is not the only way of developing knowledge at locality. New knowledge can be born without new events of practice, but it can also be created by reconsideration of what we have already learned from our practice. We learn from each piece of information that we gather, but we also learn from combining those pieces. Astronomical numbers can result from such combinations.

Why Do General Laws Often Fail to Work at a Locality, While Action Research Addresses Local Issues Successfully?

General laws fail at a locality if they do not adapt to particular local conditions. Abstract general laws must be interpreted into a local reality. The power of interpretation comes from Chigen, to which action research contributes by fostering the accumulation of tacit and articulated knowledge in context. Lewin's framing of this problem reflects his wisdom. "These laws [which researchers have identified through traditional sciences that they believe govern our practice in general] do not tell what conditions exist locally, at a given place at a given time. In other words, the laws don't do the job of diagnosis that has to be done locally. Neither do laws prescribe the strategy for change" (1946, 44). Instead of aiming at universal theories that we are very unlikely to discover, Lewin suggests that we rely on local knowledge as our starting source.

This condition has apparently overwhelmed the capabilities of the traditional social sciences. "In many fields of social science, including education, there is the sense that we have fragmented and abstracted the human experience in such a way that we no longer understand it as it is embedded in life itself" (Carson, 1990, 172). We may call this a problem of decontextualization from the local reality. General or abstract knowledge cannot adequately explain the whole situation of a given locality. Theories are always incomplete, and practice situations are never fully explained by them.

On the other hand, action research, which is grounded in location, can yield more success. Action research begins with a "felt need" of the practitioner and is concerned with questions that arise from the everyday life of practice, expressed in a language that emanates from practice (Pedretti & Hodson, 1995, 476). Action research utilizes the "tacit knowledge" and "local theory" of people in a given context throughout the whole process of a practice (Hendry, 1996). And eventually the whole results of action research are interpreted back into the improvement of a locality.

We might say that action research begins and ends with locality. In this sense its structure is a closed system. Of course, action researchers learn from external sources and publish their finding for a general audience. However, these are subsidiary functions. This contrasts with traditional sciences, which start with particularity and ends with generality in basic research, or start with generality and end with particularity in applied research. In either case, generality occupies the superior position. Action research and traditional sciences are quite distinct in this regard.

It is obvious to all of us that life is constantly changing. The world itself is changing all the time; accordingly each particular point is also permanently transforming. This is another reason that any theory or general knowledge fails to work at a local reality. Sooner or later, endlessly shifting local reality outmodes general knowledge. In contrast, action research, with its cyclic procedure, keeps fine-tuned to the ever-changing local conditions.

The above sections have alluded to four features of locality—complexity, context, particularity, and constant change—which prevent general laws from being smoothly applied in a location. General laws may not develop sufficiently to adapt to all complexities. General laws may never fully encompass the exact details of context and particularity, nor predict an ever-changing course of events. Therefore, general laws inevitably fail to some degree in local application. The solution to this problem comes from a person or persons at the site using the principles of action research, knowingly or not. Persons with high Chigen, knowledgeable in both local affairs and global principles, can effectively interpret general laws for local application.

There is yet another interesting feature of locality. Polanyi (1958, 55) explains the phenomenon of focal in contrast to subsidiary awareness. "When we use a hammer to drive in a nail," he says, "we attend to both nail and hammer, but in a different way . . . I have a subsidiary awareness of the feeling in the palm of my hand which is merged into my focal awareness of my driving in the nail." We cannot see the world from all places at once, but usually only from our locality. Thus our focal awareness has a two-fold limitation. It is constrained by our locality. We are physically bound to one location at a time, even though such a condition can sometimes be an advantage. The other constraint is that usually we can focus on only one thing at a time in order to gain a kind of knowledge that is readily put into words and used in our thinking and communication. We call it *articulate* knowledge.

There is another kind of knowledge that we may gain even through subsidiary awareness: *tacit* knowledge. We can turn our focus to innumerable things, but usually only one at a time. We can obtain rich articulate information only at the focal point and scarce or no such information at the subsidiary points. While I am rewriting my dissertation into this book, my attention is mainly directed to one passage or section at a time. The content, which comes from examination of my previous writing, also comes from one focal point at a time. The rest of the manuscript falls into subsidiary awareness. It is true that occasionally a passage or several passages of the subsidiary part may come into my focal awareness, as related to parts under current focus. Generally it is rare for such subsidiary awareness to supercede focal awareness. Therefore, the knowledge that helps my revision mainly comes from my focal passages. However, the subsidiary part functions as a backdrop against which I am examining the appropriateness of the current focal passage.

Focusing is a matter of will. A practitioner can develop a unique view based on the information that comes from one focal point, but such a fixation excludes articulate information that can be obtained through other foci. In fact, we can redirect our attention at any time to any point that we choose—imaginary or real. There may be no inaccessible points of focus in what we know and in what we see and notice; also we are capable of correlating information that has come to us serially from one focal point at a time. But we are still unable to focus, at a time, all the phenomena, or even more than an extremely small portion of the total phenomena, which make up a practice.

As action researchers work, their Chigen is accumulating knowledge particular to the location and focus of their practice. It is important for this knowledge to remain contextual. Decontextualized knowledge is like a letter without an address: useless because it cannot be delivered anywhere. The process of obtaining contextual knowledge is probably not automatic. Accurate contextual knowledge depends on careful and conscious effort relating one focal point with others either within or without the locality. As a result of this laborious effort, feelings and physical abilities and all the other attributes of personhood go through changes that help a practitioner's Chigen become empowered to carry out practice more successfully. Locality grounds the practitioner in the particularity that molds personality and is the wellspring of tacit and articulated knowledge. Locality also reflects that the contents of Chigen are always changing. Ideas are organized and reorganized, and knowledge is continuously upgraded.

At the conclusion of this chapter, it is important for us to remember the high status that local knowledge should be given. Local knowledge often plays an even more crucial part in our lives than general knowledge, though it is unwise to separate the two in practice. We have seen how and why general knowledge alone fails to solve local problems. In our educational systems, we should teach students how to enrich and refine their local knowledge so that they may become successful practitioners in their own field. Action research can play an important role in such an endeavor. Some findings suggest that we can introduce action research as a learning mode for children to enrich and refine their Chigen (e. g., Connolly & Ennew, 1996, 141-143).

Questions & Activities for Better Understanding

> The following questions and suggestions are intended to stimulate further thinking. It may not be productive to follow them in a rigid manner. The readers are encouraged to modify questions/suggestions or create new questions/suggestions so that they can engage in truly meaningful thinking and learning.

1. How did you feel and do you feel now of the importance of local knowledge? Why does local knowledge deserve more attention in action research? How can you learn endlessly from a local point? Choose a practice that you are engaged in periodically and you feel is important. Record your performance in that practice for 10 minutes. Sometime later, repeat least one more time. Reflect on the record and find out how each recording reveals some unique aspects of your practice.

2. Why do general laws fail to function appropriately in a specific local situation? How can action research remedy this problem? List any number of useful general ideas that help learners learn effectively. Develop a mini-curriculum based on these ideas. Are these ideas necessary and sufficient to develop an optimal curriculum? If they are not sufficient, what kind of knowledge is lacking there? What kind of action research may help gather relevant information to fill the gap?

3. Why does decontextualized knowledge fail to work at a certain locality? Consider the following generic example and think about a more particular case. John tries Method A at his practice and it works very well. So he shares Method A with Emily. She applies it at her place without knowing much about how John implemented that method. Emily's implementation turns out to be a total failure.

4. Describe briefly typical activities of your practice. For each activity, identify the points that you are satisfied with and those that you are not satisfied with. Why do you feel that way? How can you improve unsatisfactory points? How does action research help you gain information concerning particular points in your practice?

5. Describe the most recent activities of your practice. Choose a few activities that you would like to focus on. Expand the descriptions of the chosen activities. Later, review and reflect on the descriptions that you have produced according to the questions and suggestions in Item 4 and Item 5 (this item). Analytically

and critically examine these descriptions. What kind of research questions may be appropriate based on the previous examination?

Chapter Three

Total Engagement in Practice

How does the bridging occur in action research? What is the process of creating local knowledge? Why does the action research process require the total involvement of the practitioner's self? This chapter will examine the inner workings of the action research experience. The process of learning through hands-on experience is not unique to action research. Such learning occurs universally in our daily experience. We may call it *experiential* learning. What is unique to action research, however, is the system by which we uncover the rich learning resource that in ordinary experience is easy to overlook.

Before proceeding with this exploration, it may be helpful to clarify what has been meant by "practice" in this book. "Practice" refers to a set of activities or actions that have a specific purpose and utility. Classroom instruction is one example of a very common practice. A statewide curriculum initiative and an international joint project to improve the quality of education are examples of large-scale practices. In principle, action research can be performed on any practice. Of course, action research does not have to be limited to education. Any of NASA's various space-projects could be regarded as a practice. If a group of factory workers want to improve their productivity by doing action research, they could see their job as practice. Or on a small scale, a regular exercise of shooting basketballs might be called practice.

Ideally a practitioner is simultaneously an action researcher. But there are various situations where that is not possible. Young practitioners are unable to do action research independently, and any practitioner starting action research for the first time requires assistance. External facilitators may need to initiate action research. Researchers from academia may join action research as participants but not fully function as practitioners. Any of these situations, where action researchers are not independent or not fully involved in the practice, implies "participation" instead of "practice" in action research. Still, advocating participation of a researcher is a significant departure from the ideal of the traditional sciences, in which a researcher is regarded as an observing bystander. Yet we must say that participation is a weaker version of practice. For this reason, the following discussion will be most meaningful for authentic practice.

The last chapter examined locality that is a somewhat static component even though that is more than a mere local point. Practice is a more complex component with additional dimensions. For example, while mere locality does not demand fixed focus, allowing attention to wander anywhere, commitment to practice does not allow attention to shift as freely. Consequently, the knowledge produced by practice is more densely concentrated around the specific experience and scarce elsewhere. This fixation of focus has both positive and negative consequences. It gives uniquely rich knowledge concerning the experience, which is essential for the improvement of practice. But it does not allow a practitioner to learn about the surrounding points, significantly limiting the findings that may contribute to the improvement of practice, since those surrounding points may also be strongly connected with the practice. For example, subsidiary issues in practice such as "John, one of my students, looks upset this morning." cannot hold the attention of a practitioner for long even if it may lead to important information to improve John's learning. Therefore, while engaged wholeheartedly in practice, administering to the entire class and teaching a subject, a teacher can not give enough attention to such information about an individual student to obtain a thoughtful answer to such a situation. Bystanders' viewpoints may be the exact opposite concerning this issue. They can turn their focus on any point for any duration of time.

Too strict a fixation is not healthy, nor is it productive, as important findings often come unexpectedly from the peripheral areas of a practice. Therefore, occasional deviations of attention have merit. Even seemingly unrelated, purely playful observations may cause a life-changing discovery. Action research benefits both from the dense information focal points provide as well as from the information of peripheral and unrelated points, which is sparse, yet more unique. How? Action research accumulates various records, and we can direct our attention when we review these records, at some convenient time, to a point in any of these information sources. In reviewing, the practitioner can freely dwell on those points mentioned in the records and also on those that can be inferred from the records. This is the freedom from rigid fixation that a bystander may enjoy, even though an on-looker's knowledge is much shallower on the particular practice situation. Such freedom releases the researcher from the demands of practice. This is why action research generates more of the diverse knowledge that can facilitate fundamental improvements than experiences themselves are able to do.

In the action research mode, practitioner can more readily pick up cases like John's and have chances to think more systematically and strategically to improve the situations.

Characteristics of Practice

The learning that occurs in practice is messy, mumbled, nonlinear, recursive, and sometimes unpredictable (Avery, 1990). These traits are quite conspicuous even to the untrained. They may be called "manifest traits" in contrast with the "tacit traits" that will be discussed later in this chapter.

Messiness

Real practice is very complex, due both to locality and to the ever-changing influences of the actions and reactions of a practitioner. Innumerable factors are constantly affecting the course of a practitioner's experience. Physical, emotional, spiritual, social, political, and many other dimensions are concurrently involved. Moreover, it is never clear how these dimensions comprise the reality of practice at the next moment.

Since in our research we are seeking for order and for a more clearly defined reality, it is tempting to ignore or reject the messiness we encounter, paying attention only to those areas where order is apparent or where we can easily impose order. But it is important to face the reality that our experience is messy and to be tolerant of this messiness and accept it positively. This does not mean that we should remain in messiness or be indifferent to it, but that we should not try to merely escape from it to the clearer portions of reality, which the majority of traditional scientists have been investigating. Such a tendency is compared to searching for a lost coin only in a well-lit spot under a street light. We should purposefully and intentionally train ourselves to handle this messiness most meaningfully. Our experience is not just complex; it is richly complex. What we first perceive as messiness often contains much relevant information valuable to our practice. If only we develop skills and a right attitude, we can tap this endless resource. Action research, with its newly acquired naturalistic or qualitative techniques, can provide us the means to undertake this challenging task.

Nonlinearity

Our practice involves many factors, and the number of those factors is changing all the time. In addition, an infinite number of other factors within and without our scope indirectly influence practice to varying degrees. As a result, our practice can not proceed in a linear fashion. Continually our action is pulled in various directions and goes off on many tangents. Of course, some portions of our work may have an approximate linearity, which case allows us , in planning, to identify a dominant factor of a specific action so that we can roughly predict the course of that action. This point will be discussed further in the next chapter. However, it is wise to be cautious about the inherent limitations in such a prediction.

Dynamism

Experience reveals that practitioners in their work settings undertake more complex syntheses of different types of input information than academics do in their research (Yeatman, 1996, 295). Practitioners' personal involvement promotes these complex syntheses, changing the course of practice and resulting in more knowledge of greater richness and depth than bystanders would obtain by observing the practice. This involvement process changes the nature of the original environment, so that even from the inside the environment is constantly being reshaped (McKernan, 1991, 24; Manicas & Secord, 1983, 403). A dynamic relationship also exists between subjective and objective conditions, and this dynamism is provoked by action (Zuber-Skerritt 1992, 68). Action not only carries focal awareness to different points in the practice, it works as a medium through which Chigen acts upon the tasks of the practice and receives responses back from these tasks. Action also works as a stimulant on the tasks so that information may be readily released from them.

Constructivism is usefully employed in explaining this situation. Reality is being constantly constructed in two different modes—in narrative and in practical action (Baillie 1996, 307). Our Chigen is constantly interacting with our practice as well as with the Chigen of others, thus producing new knowledge, new perspectives, and eventually a new and refined Chigen. Zuber-Skerritt sheds further light on this process. To know an object is to act on it so as to transform it. And through these transformations, we grasp the mechanism of how they occur. To know, therefore, is to produce the object dynamically; but to reproduce, it is also necessary to know how to produce, and this is why knowledge derives from the entire action, not merely from its figurative aspects. The structure of memory is a system that learns through an active interaction with its environment, rather than a passive build up of stimulus-response connections (Zuber-Skerritt 1992, 69-78). Knowledge that acquired from a book or a paper also remains passive before it goes through the refining fire of reality in practice. Active knowledge is only attainable through active labor. A willful and intentional attitude is also a prerequisite of such knowledge acquisition.

As constructivism indicates, the reality we construct of a practice is produced as we act on the practice. Likewise, the quality and focus of the knowledge produced through practice strongly depends on the quality and focus of the chosen action. The knowledge obtained through a bystander's observation will never be as comprehensive as that of an actor in practice. Thoughtful actions produce high quality knowledge that can directly improve our practice. Speaking metaphorically, action is a window through which we can observe and learn much about practice.

Unpredictability

As we have already seen in the section on nonlinearity, we cannot exactly predict the course of actions in practice. No single theory can fully explain a practice. It is easy to account for this unpredictability by examining messiness, nonlinearity, and dynamism. It may be wise not to spend great effort and time for prediction that may be wasted because of a change in circumstances. The Trukese, a group of Pacific Islanders, navigate by breaking a path to their destination down into many small steps. Each step has a small goal to reach, and the course of the work is adjusted and readjusted according to the outcome of each step. If a complete chart of the sea was available—along with the necessary technology, we could advantageously navigate according to a grand plan. Yet since our practice is still uncharted, we must, like the Trukese, rely on small incremental steps.

How does such an approach work? If we were leaving for a voyage without a chart, we would begin by sailing toward the first visible target. While sailing toward the first target, we would see the second; while aiming for the second, we would sight the third etc. Thus we could go further and further, from island to island.

This approach well represents how action research works in our practice. It may not be difficult to set a rough first target to improve our practice. The second and third targets are not visible at the beginning. They can only come into our sight after carrying out action toward the first target. The objectives and plans of action research should continually be adjusted throughout the action research cycle. Action research does not exclude a grand plan or a longitudinal goal as long as it fits the purpose of the action research. Such a grand plan will undoubtedly require frequent revisions to adapt to the ever-changing situations of action research. In action research, everything may and should be ever changing. The scope, methodology, and skills of the research, as well as the plan and objectives for improvement, are constantly changing or developing. Above all, practitioners themselves are improving their performance and character.

How can we make best use of such unpredictable circumstances? First, grand plans and longitudinal goals are not to be excluded from action research; they are even desirable if they are sufficiently flexible and tentative. They may balance the tendency of action researchers to focus on overly narrow and particular points of practice. However, the majority of the practitioner's attention should be on moment-to-moment concerns of the local circumstances. Second, if instead of investing time and effort on the search for universal principles and laws we focus on describing and interpreting local phenomena, our action research should be more productive. Even though we cannot always predict or prescribe our course of action, we can still improve our practice and understand it better when we describe and interpret it. By doing so, we can deal with unpredictable situations more meaningfully through the enrichment of our Chigen.

During the last century two major research methodologies emerged: phenomenology and hermeneutics. Phenomenology guides us in the search of the essences in practice. Hermeneutics teaches us how to interpret and reinterpret the meaning of our experience and existence. An integrative approach, hermeneutic phenomenology, advocated by Max van Manen (1986, 1990, 1991b, 1991a), provides an especially powerful means to investigate meaning in our local situations.

Multi-dimensionality and the Total Involvement of the Self

People understand themselves and their environment, and anticipate future events by constructing tentative models or personal theories and by evaluating these theories against personal criteria based on the success of this prediction and control. This process of construction involves many dimensions of our existence. Such understanding requires the active, creative, rational, emotional, intentional and pragmatic construction of reality (Zuber-Skerritt 1993, 53). Similarly, action research involves our whole being: feelings, self-concepts (e. g., metacognition, self-belief, self-esteem, self-efficacy, etc.), and many other faculties of our personhood. Deep learning occurs in action research when the reality of practice heavily touches multiple facets of personhood. If we can create such contact intentionally and willfully, our action research will generate valuable knowledge. We cannot improve things without affecting them. Likewise, we cannot effectively gain knowledge without being affected by it. Otherwise, what we acquire is an "armchair theory." Such interactivity may not always be easy or comfortable. Practice, especially when it is innovative, often becomes "a process in which anxiety, conflict, and occasional exhaustion are guaranteed" (Sands & Drake 1996, 77). We know well through our experiences that sacrifices are required for a great accomplishment. An Asian proverb "Koketsu ni irazunba koji o ezu" (You cannot catch a tiger's cub without getting into its den) and a western equivalent "Nothing ventured, nothing gained" describe this principle.

People seem to develop a number of fallacies about our self-concept. Self-knowledge is commonly given, at best, secondary status in our knowledge base, yet is a crucial active component of the base. We often believe erroneously that we know ourselves well. It was only after some years of living in a foreign country that my family came to realize how little we had known about Japanese culture when we were still in our home country. If I ask at the beginning of a semester my students in my college freshmen course on intercultural communication to describe their own culture, the majority of them cannot do it well. If we look back on how our self-knowledge has developed, we find that the process consists of many experiences in which we faced a different self or engaged in serious self-reflection that was probably affected by others. We cannot expect that valid self-knowledge will develop without conflicts and struggles with others.

Action research helps us know ourselves better. To illustrate, I will use a personal experience that I will elaborate further in Chapter Six. Such knowledge occurred very unexpectedly. When my family was enthusiastically engaged in a family game in a winter vacation, I decided to do a little action research to improve my performance. As I recorded my own and the others' performances and scores in a log, then analyzed and reflected on the data, I began to realize that the data contained not just information about our performances, but that it also offered insight into our characteristics. I was surprised by the degree to which the data revealed my own personality.

Experiential learning begins with the self-concept or self-image of the learner (Hendry 1996, 627). It is desirable, if circumstances may allow, to monitor our personal traits at any stage of practice, because such a small investment may bring a large return. Personal growth through action research is one of the quickest and surest ways that guarantee the improvement of a practice. We may wonder, "Do I attempt this action research to achieve personal growth, or do I improve myself in order to improve my practice?" When we are totally engaged in a practice, it is hard to distinguish between these two processes; they happen concurrently and complementarily.

To provide for the multi-variable multi-layer conditions of practice, action research is necessarily pluralistic in focus. Existing positivistic theories are insufficient and too simplistic for this pluralistic function. Positivistic approaches are weak, especially because they disregard or shut out from the research process the human elements that are essential for successful practice. Practice happens simultaneously at various layers. Feelings, interest, will, belief, and all the other faculties of a human being must be under good control for successful practice. Knowledge is created at all the faculties of a human being while practitioners are whole-heartedly tackling with their practice.

Knowledge is often produced in reflection as well. Reflection examines and expands the all kinds of knowledge that a practice continuously produces. Thus, the knowledge that action research can produce is very versatile. Reflection involves insight, feelings and intuition, as well as logical deduction (Anderson 1994, 26). One of the unique characteristics of action research is that it produces meta-faculty knowledge (the knowledge about these human faculties, e.g., meta-cognitive knowledge), and action research can utilize such knowledge more appropriately than do traditional sciences (Rist 1982, x). Such meta-knowledge helps a practitioner monitor each faculty so that it functions appropriately and has harmonious relationships with the other faculties.

Feelings, one aspect of human faculties, may serve as an example applicable to other faculties as well. The knowledge coming from any practice is encumbered with feelings and values. Our personal signatures are imprinted on our practice because our feelings are involved. We should not disregard but welcome the inevitable involvement of our feelings in our practice. Feelings underlie any intentional action: to promote or impede, with weak or strong association. The role of feelings is decisive.

The Role of Feelings

It is not the purpose of this book to discuss each of the human faculties individually. It suffices to choose one major faculty: feelings. To best generalize to the other faculties, we use the broadest definition of feeling, which includes senses, signals sent from senses, sensation, sentiment, emotion, affection, sensitivity, passion, awareness, consciousness, intuitive knowledge, and so on. It is not an exaggeration to say that feelings affect all phases of action research. As already noted action research begins with felt need. Feelings convey information, they motivate the production of new knowledge, and they form the basis of our evaluation of information. Feelings connect us to our inner knowledge or meta-faculty knowledge and to our knowledge of the external world (Peake 1992, 103). Feelings serve not only to promote action but also to guide movement or change. Thus we learn and grow as we experience feelings, and in fact it is what we feel that enables us to learn and grow. Moreover, feelings are the most authentic representation of our inner self; we know others better by eliciting their feelings about different situations than by observing their behavior (Gianotti 1994, 58).

Certain functions of feelings may be more important than others. Consciousness is the central faculty of human beings which is fundamentally involved in personal transformation (Baillie 1996, 305). At the center of human experience, there is consciousness, which is evoked both by the inner workings of a human being and by practice. A variety of other feelings on the periphery direct those inner workings, either clouding or intensifying consciousness.

Feelings are crucial in making judgments (Hargreaves 1997, 16). A free decision-making process starts with the feeling of preference. While we examine each alternative, we experience various feelings such as anxiety, excitement, and peace, which help us select a suitable option. At each significant junction of a practice, feelings signal whether we should go ahead or should stop there to take a different course of action. Thus, the feelings with their work can be one of the most powerful contributions of action research to practitioners (Baskett & Hill 1990, 32).

Action research sometimes influences practitioners' feelings more than thinking processes (Baskett & Hill 1990, 253). And those feelings affect knowledge development in unique ways as the knowledge becomes personalized. Thus personal knowledge is never free from "biases" and "skewness" as we discussed in a previous chapter (Reason 1993, 1262). In action research we see these two descriptors, which are usually used negatively, in a new and positive light. "Uniqueness" and "distinctiveness" are additional descriptors for these same characteristics. We cannot separate them. Likewise we cannot separate practitioners' thinking in action research from their feelings and attitudes, their being and their sense of self (Dadds 1993, 229). Therefore, if we look at this phenomenon holistically, we should say that the integration of emotionality in the action research process is not weakness, but enrichment and strength (Chisholm 1990, 253). Once a change takes place in feelings, the effects are often prompt and far-reaching.

Tacit Knowledge

Much of our knowledge is tacit and cannot be articulated (Polanyi 1958). Tacit knowledge cannot be adequately explained verbally because it pertains to nonverbal information. It is carried in our bodies, as in the process of riding a bicycle. Verbal direction and knowledge can help us improve our tacit knowledge, or use it to better purpose, or transfer it from one realm to another. My daughter's effort to learn a hand-wheel in her gymnastics lesson, which heavily involves tacit knowledge, is greatly helped by the coach's verbal instructions and by model performances on which she bases her subsequent practice. The verbal instruction helps her develop articulate knowledge, and the modeling and practice give tacit knowledge that assists her to connect the articulate knowledge with the performances so that the articulate knowledge transfers to action and guides her exercise. Articulate knowledge does not exist on the fringe of tacit knowledge; rather it is embedded in it, like ships of articulate knowledge floating on an ocean of tacit knowledge. However, this does not devalue articulate knowledge, because articulate knowledge is the only form that can be examined by logic and it comprises the raw materials with which we think and reason. Yet we must realize that if we peel back the skin-deep layer of articulate knowledge, we will find much tacit knowledge.

Through interactions with our environment, limitless tacit knowledge is gained, but only the points on which we focus generate articulate knowledge. For example, if intercultural communication is our practice, one form of interaction would probably be dialogue with a foreigner. It is obvious that communication is much more than exchange of words. Any verbal exchange is accompanied by the constant flow of varied emotions. In order to comprehend intended meanings accurately, we must pay careful attention to facial expressions, body language, and the context within which the dialogue generates a particular meaning. It is ordinarily quite apparent that what the words communicate is only a tip of an iceberg.

Objectivity

Even though much attention is turned to subjectivity, objectivity is not unimportant in action research. At any stage of action research it is appropriate and beneficial to check the objectivity of our knowledge. We can obtain objectivity in various ways, as we do in the traditional sciences: collecting information from multiple independent sources, performing controlled experiments, following statistical procedures, and so forth. In addition, objectivity in action research is increased when practitioners share and discuss their interpretations of the issues with others (Hustler et al. 1986, 9). "The White House is in Washington, DC" is an objective statement. The law of gravity influences any object on this earth. Aging is inevitable for any human being. These pieces of objective knowledge cannot differ through interpretation. When objectivity is ensured, knowledge becomes general, transferable, robust, stable, consistent, and trustworthy. Objective testing is applicable over a significant portion of action research.

However, human action and growth are largely rooted in how we perceive situations and take personal meaning from them. Therefore, objectivity is not as significant as it is in non-human phenomena. To attain objectivity we detach knowledge from locality by extracting or abstracting ideas from their complex context. When we require objectivity from our knowledge, the knowledge becomes neutral, but at the same time the value judgment concerning the knowledge is set aside. Loss of personal meaning, which is the power of knowledge to prompt people to action, is in the price that is paid for the objectification of phenomena. Hence objectivity, if it is imposed mindlessly and if it oppresses subjectivity, is a significant impediment to the natural human development of practitioners.

How does action research see the objective knowledge that has been so well established in other fields of research? Action research does not deny the value of such knowledge, but it cannot utilize it directly. Since it has been abstracted from local reality, it has to be reinterpreted into the particular local context. Admittedly, this is easier said than done. For example, when a practitioner comes up with two methods (Method A and B) to deal with a certain activity, he or she can gain objective knowledge about the comparative effectiveness of these two methods based on an empirical study. Such a study typically requires standardization and control, where abstraction and decontextualization are inevitable. After the study, the action researcher may conclude that Method A is more effective than Method B. In what way? We can safely say that Method A is more effective in a certain controlled procedure. Is it objective knowledge? Yes, but by being objective it is somewhat detached from the complex local situation of that activity. Therefore, when the action researcher/practitioner implements Method A in the real activity, he or she must make many adjustments. The knowledge about these adjustments does not come with that objective knowledge. A successful implementation of objective knowledge, therefore, imposes two different challenges. The detached and decontextualized objective knowledge must be re-transplanted into a particular local context. Secondly, it must be continuously readjusted to the ever-changing local reality of the practice. It requires thoughtful practitioners with rich experiences with the locality to accomplish such a successful interpretation. The practitioners' Chigen must be fully developed for such success.

Subjectivity

Consciousness, agency, intention, and action are defining components of social behavior. They are crucial components of action research as well, and it is obvious that all of these factors are grounded in subjectivity. Subjectivity pervades the whole course of action research. Subjectivity is an aspect of knowledge that is both conscious and unconscious, which expresses our identity as human agents (Errigton 1993, 31). Subjectivity is the personal signature on any work. We might say that the very essence of action research is to raise the subjectivity in practitioners from a low and crude form to a more refined and well-examined form. In other words, an action researcher is an acting agent who starts with subjectivity and refines it throughout the process of action research (MicNiff 1988, 50).

In action research, practitioners are active seekers and negotiators of meaning, both world producers and social products (Zuber-Skerritt 1993, 51). The object of a study is at the same time a subject who owns the action research and decides the course of action for producing new knowledge. Action research uses subjectivity and objectivity in a unique blend. Moreover, it is subjectivity that promotes the most important processes of action. Then how can action research claim validity while it has a strong subjective tendency as opposed to the traditional sciences?

To answer this question, we must first examine the definition of validity. Traditionally, validity has been one of the central issues of research, and this importance has not diminished over time. However, during the last few decades there has been a drastic shift in the way of looking at it. The qualitative research orientations have increasingly been recognized. Guba and Lincoln (1985) did a most comprehensive work that truly represents these orientations. A decade later, Watkins and Brooks (1994) developed a unique set of criteria for action research, inspired by Guba and Lincoln (1985). Table 1 outlines these two sets of criteria for validity. As all of these approaches including traditional positivistic approaches have a common ground to establish the truthfulness of their findings, their differences must be carefully analyzed, as they are easily erroneously exaggerated. Therefore, we need not assume that the quite different wording in this table implies the demise of the traditional criteria in the new epistemologies. Instead, we should consider these criteria as new interpretations of the common ground premises on which the traditional criteria are also based.

The Two New Ways to Look at Validity
(The wording was modified by the author.)

Naturalistic Inquiry (Guba & Lincoln)	Action Research (Watkins & Brooks)
Trustworthiness/Credibility To what extent can we make people trust the findings? To what extent do the findings truthfully fit the local context?	**Skillfulness** To what extent can action researchers develop skills for both practice and research so that they can make the findings work in the local context?
Transferabiligy/Applicability To what extent can the findings work at different local contexts and for different practitioners.	**Relevancy/Usability** To what extent do the findings fit the needs of the local context?
Dependability/Consistency To what extent can the findings be repeated with the similar contexts and practitioners?	**System Competency** To what extent can the findings support the systemic or holistic development of the practice?
Confirmability/Neutrality To what extent can the findings be determined by the practitioners and the context of the inquiry, not by the biases of the research?	**Normative/Consistency** To what extent are the research procedures guided by the principles of action research? To what extent do the practitioners grow? Is their practice improved as generally expected by action research?

Table 1

Free Agency

Agency is the innate freedom that is given to every human being to behave according to his or her choice in any contingency. Behavior is shaped by reinforcement contingencies, and once individuals can modify these, the power of contingencies as an independent force is lost (Secord 1984, 29). This contingent-independent choice is well illustrated in an old saying, "You can lead a horse to water but you can't make it drink." Laws of the land can bind our behavior but cannot control our thought against our will. Humans are self-determining. Humans differ from objects in their capacity to self-reflect, to diagnose their own problems, and to generate knowledge (Susman & Evered 1978, 586). Agency should be fully active, allowing us to interpret—in our unique way—the local situations, and based on this interpretation we make decisions. Therefore, it is not an exaggeration to say that there is no such a thing as non-interpreted experience in the world of action (Manicas & Secord 1983, 410). Moreover, agents interpret the meaning of their own actions (Zuber-Skerritt 1992, 78). Our practice is full of meaningful and intentional actions where agency plays the vital role. Agency is the soil from which human competence germinates.

Subjectivity appropriately grows only when a person's agency is endorsed. Since every human being already has free agency, the question is how to secure, respect, and utilize that agency in action research. As demonstrated in the chapter on ownership (Chapter One), this is not necessarily an easy task. If you are facilitating action research, you need a holistic understanding of human nature, without which you cannot truly secure the agency of practitioners. Additionally, unless you have fully lived action research yourself by exercising your own free agency, you will lead as a blind man leads the blind. This is not the blindness of some people who practice action research naturally without realizing it. Since none of the five components of action research is the exclusive domain of action research, some people might be doing action research accidentally. I have encountered many examples of people I would classify as action researchers in my reading about the educational history of Japan, where action research was scarcely known decades ago. Those who live the five action research principles without noticing doing so could mindfully lead others to be a truly free agent in their endeavor. My main observation, though, is that we have not fully exercised or facilitated agency in action research.

Since free agency does not come with any prescribed code of behavior, a person must make choices and take initiative in action. Many people find difficulty in choosing their own course of action. They expect to be told how to do their task. Some are afraid of making decisions. Learning how to become a more independent agent may be a slow process, requiring intense nurture. Do we dare to ask such a task of our educational system? This question will be explored in a later section of this text.

In general, action research should secure the agency of a practitioner as much as the situation allows. It is possible to disregard agency and still have a superficial form of action research, but a fundamental and true change in a practitioner does not occur if agency, including the appropriate level of ownership, is not bestowed. The more ownership is given to practitioners, the more freedom they gain to exercise their agency. Generally action research respects the agency of practitioners far more than the traditional scientific research. It is important to note that creating an environment in which a practitioner may be able to fully exercise his or her agency does not guarantee that a practitioner will take advantage of that freedom and do high quality action research. Whether or not a practitioner does action research wholeheartedly is totally his or her decision, which is what agency is all about. You cannot force action research, you can only facilitate it, and especially sensitive care must be taken in this process.

Refined Subjectivity

Many aspects of subjectivity have been treated in previous sections. Therefore, those points are now reviewed to further study the process of refining subjective judgment. We have contrasted aspects of objectivity and subjectivity in action research. These are both distinct and complementary, but subjectivity is emphasized in action research. We delineated how agency makes subjectivity essential in knowledge production. When our agency is respectfully acknowledged, and when we are fully aware of various possibilities to exert it, subjectivity is ready to be cultivated.

Granting such acknowledgement often means taking risks, as we experience in nurturing teenagers. Accommodating to their demands increases their freedom and independence, which often tests our patience. We also know that such risk taking is the only way they will grow personally. Practitioners' subjectivity or personal judgement grows according to the same principle—taking risks, making mistakes, analyzing situations, and learning from them. Subjectivity is refined through interaction and struggle with the reality of the practice.

The pursuit of objectivity also contributes greatly to this refining process. My son's violin practice, which in its early stages had made me plug my ears, gradually improved due to three things: practicing scales, frequently tuning by a keyboard, and playing with a metronome. Those three external measures helped my son's internal skill development. Our subjectivity is always prone to deviation and bias. Therefore, objectivity check is necessary in adjusting our course of action. Piaget, one of the greatest psychologists of the 20th century, uniquely described this developmental process. He maintained that any object in practice is gradually discovered in its objective properties by a decentering process (decentration) that frees knowledge of its subjective illusions. It is from this same interaction that the subject, by discovering and conquering the object, organizes his or her actions into a coherent system that constitutes the operations of his or her intelligence and his or her thought (Piaget 1977, 31). As humans we are inevitably bound to locality and are self-centered by nature. To outgrow such limitations, we need some consistent external measure against which we can check our internal measure—subjectivity.

At this point we can name a few principles which foster refined subjectivity. First, our subjectivity must be guided by free agency in as active and free an exploration of our practice as possible. Second, our ever-developing subjectivity must be refined through continuous confrontation with the indomitable objective reality. Therefore, we should proactively employ those external measures to examine our subjectivity as much as possible. Third, our subjectivity is also examined through dialogues with others. It is very beneficial to involve "critical" friends in an action research project. And additionally our subjectivity is cultivated through reflection, in which memory or recorded facts function as a touchstone. Since subjectivity is the central part of Chigen, it is wise to direct enough effort to this refining process so that Chigen develops efficiently.

Although action research can be employed merely as a tool or technique that does not deal with intricate subjectivity issues, it is wise to better understand them in order to fully count on the "being"—a perpetual powerhouse for ideas and actions. More proactively, if we can somehow maintain and upgrade the integrity of each action researcher as a human being and the community of his or her associates, action research should become more meaningful and far-reaching. The next section will explore another dimension of action research that is yet to be studied systematically. Since there is no standardized framework by which to discuss this topic, I will draw ideas from my personal experiences and thought and present them as a particular case that should be examined by many others to establish a universal framework for this issue—spirituality.

Morality and Spirituality

Next to divine guidance, I believe, refined subjectivity is the most reliable source upon which to base personal life changing decisions. In action research, in comparison with the traditional sciences, an important shift is being proposed from reliance on method as the basis of knowing to reliance on the human person and the human community (Reason 1993, 1259). I feel strongly that I can rely on the personal witness of trustworthy persons with whom I have an enduring relationship more than on a physical evidence that I often cannot see in its entirety. It is true that even good people can give erroneous information, so I have to examine carefully the context of their assurance and the grounds on which they have come to their conclusions. However, once I am convinced of the trustworthiness of both the person and his or her statement, I would trust my life with that message. In contrast, physical evidences, which may be only partially available, are often misleading. They can be presented in such a way that they give off a distorted image.

For example, I have seen how statistics can be used to mislead. The next three figures show how different visual representations based on the same statistics can lead to different impressions. Figure 2 is the trend of Stock A during the last 18 years. Probably most of us feel negative about the company since it has performed poorly over a long period. Figure 3 shows only the last three years of the trend. Although this truncated graph may make us suspicious, the trend does suggest growth. Figure 4 has manipulated the same three years to suggest rapid growth.

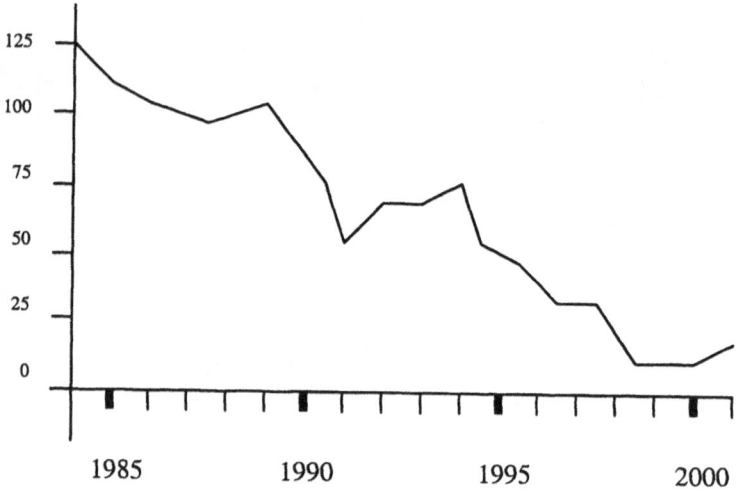

Figure 2

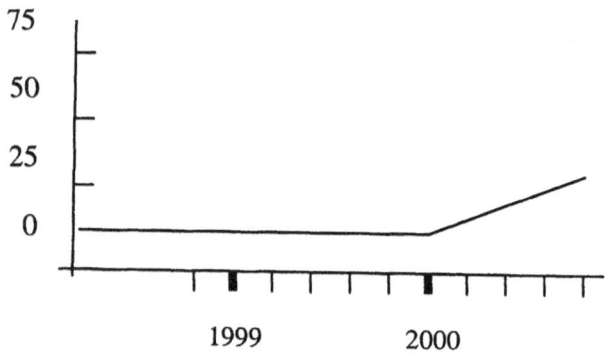

Figure 3

Manipulated Rapid Growth

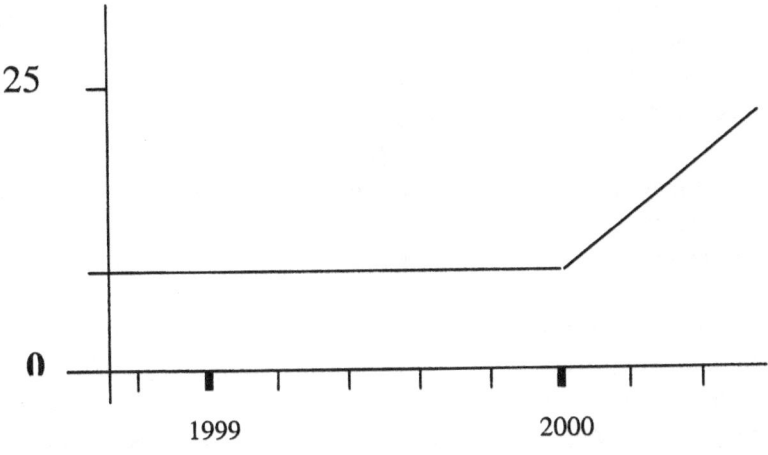

Figure 4

On the other hand, the same presentation may give different people different impressions. Some people may find favorable evidence for investment in the downward trend of Figure 2. They may expect even a higher profit from this stock than from other high performers when they sense that the current stock market evaluates the company much lower than it truly deserves. This simple illustration is sufficient to demonstrate how even statistics, the most common tool in representing objective knowledge, can be so differently presented and interpreted according to objectives, foci, and perspectives. Of course, this illustration does not disregard the general utility of objectivity and statistics.

Wrestling within the objective reality of a practice is a refining process for our subjectivity. Conversation with others also examines our subjectivity from an outside viewpoint. Subjectivity trained this way is trustworthy. Although such trustworthiness is field dependent (trustworthy in one thing but perhaps not in another) because of their extensive experience in their field I often follow the advice of my mentors over the apparent implications of physical evidence I have collected. Because of their greater experience I trust that their picture of a given situation is more complete than mine.

I believe that it is appropriate to point out here one particular dimension of subjectivity—spirituality—a key element that distinctly affects the outcomes of action research. By "spirituality" I mean the attributes that are beyond the physical and cognitive spheres of our existence. Those attributes make people ethical and trustworthy. Without an assurance of minimum spirituality in action researchers, we cannot trust the validity of their findings. In practice, which is supposedly desirable and appropriate for both the practitioners and the society, they can perform more effectively and productively in such a way as to amplify the wellness of themselves and the society when they maintain a higher spirituality. Unfortunately, however, our society at large does not necessarily foster spirituality among its people; on the contrary, it harbors the leanings toward corruption and permits such pitfalls and snares as can annihilate the spiritual growth. Such a tendency can be found all over the world and throughout human history.

Currently, education is increasingly secularized and weakening its inspiring power to uplift people, as the fabric of society—family—is gradually disintegrating and losing the capability to foster spirituality in children, and increasing corruption and immorality among political leaders are desensitizing the public conscience. Then, how can we, as practitioners, nurture spirituality not only in ourselves but also in those who are somehow related with us while we are engaged in our practice?

Since I can hardly find any systematic study of this issue, based on which I can device strategies to maintain or promote spirituality in our community, I would like to reflect on my own up-bringing to seek for a lead on this matter. When I discuss the spiritual roots below, I do not claim that mine are unique, as there are many respectable spiritual root systems of organized religion and of personal belief in the world. And since this is largely a matter of metaphysics, I will not attempt to prove my position either. I will simply present mine as one of the particular cases.

There are three major associations that have mainly affected my spirituality besides my personal inclination and experiences: family, friends and associates (including those found in books, music, performing art, etc.), and religious affiliation. How can we strengthen those associations so that they can, in turn, nurture our spirituality as well as our children? When we are wholeheartedly engaged in action research (as I illustrate in my episode in the last chapter), unexpectedly and repeatedly we encounter the spiritual reality of our self. The accounts of any action researcher that document those moments should provide useful data that enable systematic studies to generate principles and guidelines to enhance our spirituality.

Meanwhile, I would like to continue my reflection on personal case to illustrate the potential that an organized religion can play a significant role to help us be more trustworthy practitioners and action researchers. Through my experiences for several years in Shinto, the Japanese original religion, and 33 years in Christianity of the Church of Jesus Christ of Latter-day Saints, I have learned that we are spiritual as well as physical, emotional, and intellectual beings. My conviction has grown through listening to thousands of testimonies of my fellow church members. I have also closely observed their lives. Very often their living examples have more eloquently born a witness to me. I have also learned that our spiritual growth is specifically dependent on how we relate ourselves with a higher spiritual being: in my case, the Savior, Jesus Christ. I do not deny the goodness of any humanistic movements and activities that are also influencing my spiritual life. However, I cannot compare such influences with that which comes from my continuous personal relationship with my Savior in terms of intensity and power. The following quotation explains how I am obtaining guidance from above concerning important issues in my personal and family life.

> You must study it out in your mind; then you must ask me if it be right, and if it is right I will cause that your bosom shall burn within you; therefore, you shall feel that it is right. But if it be not right you shall have no such feelings, but you shall have a stupor of thought that shall cause you to forget the thing which is wrong. (Doctrine and Covenants 9:8-9, The Church of Jesus Christ of Latter-day Saints)

Through many experiences I have learned this promise is true. As it tells us, first we must do our best to figure out our problems; then we are qualified to present our tentative solution before God. The guidance comes through two channels—our mind and feelings. Occasionally we receive unattainable ideas through the former channel if we are worthy or our situation is appropriate for such a privilege. We often feel very warm and peaceful feelings, as assurance that what we ask is right, and uneasy feelings when what we ask for is inappropriate. I know that what I have explained so far concerning my spiritual examination is a very personal, individual process. Yet I believe that similar experiences are happening to many in this global society, no matter what religion or philosophy they believe or espouse, if they are listening to their conscience.

I believe that my God, who is also known as the God of Abraham, the God of Isaac, and the God of Jacob, "inviteth them [the children of men] all to come unto him and partake of his goodness; and he denieth none that come unto him, black and white, bond and free, male and female; and he remembereth the heathen; and all are alike unto God, both Jew and Gentile" (II Nephi 26:33, The Book of Mormon). I believe the divine guidance and the "voice of conscience" have the same roots. In the world history there are many inspiring stories of those who assiduously followed this voice of conscience. Socrates, Confucius,

George Washington, Johann Heinrich Pestalozzi, Leo Tolstoy, Mahatma Gandhi, Albert Schweitzer, and Mother Teresa are just a few of the countless whose lives have edified the world with their ideas and examples.

The "voice of conscience" tells us to be honest, kind, mindful, fair, obedient, humble, meek, compassionate, and loving. It also tells us not to kill, steal, despise, and take advantage of others' weaknesses. It encourages us not to be cruel, indifferent, selfish, greedy, and proud. Unfortunately sciences themselves do not guide us to those virtues. Sciences only serve as tools for us to better understand the phenomena pertaining to our physical world, psychological world, and potentially spiritual world. Sciences do not invite or encourage us to cherish any particular virtue because they must be value-neutral to claim their universality and generalizability. It is religions and philosophies that lead us to those virtues. Thus we need to have spiritual roots through which we can nurture our spirituality.

These positive attributes that we develop by following our conscience are the crucial basis for judging the validity of the knowledge action researchers produce. We cannot trust the report of those who obviously lack those positive attributes since such a report reflects their inappropriate personal inclination. As a bent mirror cannot reflect an image correctly, a crooked person tends to distort a wholesome truth about his or her own experience because his or her perspective is crooked and the experience can be likewise. Elliot, after leading the teacher-researcher movement in the Great Britain for more than fifteen years, said, "The time may have arrived for facilitators of reflective practice to stop using the term 'action research.' I found myself trying to express the idea which is referred to in different ways. I have started to talk about reflective practice as a 'moral science'" (1991b, 52). Without moral or spiritual foundation of action researchers, the knowledge they produce may actually prove to be detrimental, rather than advantageous, to our society. However, little scientific study has been done about how to develop morality and spirituality; hopefully there will be advancements in this area in the near future.

Relevance

It is in practice itself that the most relevant knowledge is produced. The standard by which we judge relevance in action research is very simple and clear: If "it works," it is relevant; if "it does not work," it is irrelevant. As in the example of my daughter's gymnastics lesson, thoughtful combination of relevant articulate knowledge (written or oral) and tacit knowledge (observation and other life experiences) produces knowledge capable of being translated to action. The knowledge produced by practice is the most meaningful for practice because it is real-life data existing in real time (Cunningham 1993, 5).

Argyris et al. point out that there is a gap between "theory-in-use" and "espoused theory" (Argyris, Putnam, & Smith 1985, 81). This gap is what makes an espoused theory irrelevant to practice, in contrast to theory-in-use, which is handling in reality. Theory-in-use, however, is often unexamined and thus is likely to be less than ideal. Argyris et al.'s contribution was to illuminate a difference that we do not usually distinguish between the two theory-types. Careful examination proves that there are many similar distinctions that we fail to make. For example, we may say that we believe one thing and yet act against that belief even when we have no intention to deceive. Espoused theory may be an ideal or goal that we have not yet reached, so that a gap is born naturally between ideal and reality. Since tacit components constitute a significant part of theory-in-use, as tacit knowledge generally prevails in practice, we hardly articulate the acting theory-in-use and recognize the gap. Practice situations generally prevent us from focusing on theory-in-use. Therefore, we must employ action research to create a space in which our minds can investigate the theory-in-use.

Argyris et al.'s idea also suggests that there are experiential and other types of irrelevance in addition to structural irrelevance. Structural irrelevance occurs systematically by our desiring something better or higher than our current conditions. This phenomenon exists in any human life, and this kind of irrelevance can work positively by promoting our practice to a higher plane.

One different type of irrelevance occurs depending on our experience or maturity of Chigen. In this type and others, irrelevance is seen differently from one person to another. One person can easily apply a novel idea in his or her practice, while another cannot see any connection between the idea and his or her practice. Some people can apply borrowed ideas more readily and aggressively either because they have a more extensive knowledge base in their practice, or because they have more extensive experience in their practice and have thus developed special skills to interpret ideas into their practice. Less experienced and less skillful people find more experiential irrelevance when they see the same idea.

There is another type of irrelevance, which can be designated *motivational irrelevance*. Lack of motivation discourages practitioners from dwelling on an idea. Even when motivation is sufficient, *attitudinal irrelevance* may prevent an idea from working in practice. Some people easily believe, embrace faith, and develop self-efficacy in applying new ideas and simply put them into action, while others are lacking these qualities.

We can reasonably surmise that the raison d'etre of action research is to attack structural irrelevance, since bridging is its mission. As the Chigen of practitioners is most likely to grow optimally through action research, experiential irrelevance should be most effectively resolved by action research. Furthermore, devoted action researchers have unequivocal advantages over traditional researchers to tackle motivational and attitudinal irrelevance.

The Relationship between Practice and Chigen

This chapter has explored a great deal about the nature and contents of Chigen. Practice is messy and so is the interior of Chigen. There is a great deal of unorganized information stored in Chigen, probably the majority of which is tacit knowledge. Personhood is the center of Chigen, and subjectivity is the center of personhood. Without proper respect for and exercise of agency, subjectivity cannot develop, and we cannot enrich and refine Chigen. Although subjectivity plays the greater role in Chigen, objective knowledge also has its place, helping to examine and refine subjectivity. All of the faculties of personhood generate unique knowledge that is particular and local, with both tacit and articulate components. This can also be said of the knowledge associated with Chigen.

The content of Chigen is much more diverse and deep than we are usually aware. Articulate knowledge exists at every corner of Chigen, pointing toward and reminding us of the tacit elements that also exist throughout Chigen. The unarticulated portion of Chigen grows larger all the time. In fact when we try to articulate one point of the tacit portion, we generate another portion of tacit knowledge at the related subsidiary points just by performing such articulation. This creates a dilemma, but it is still beneficial to become more aware of what is contained in such a reservoir of knowledge.

The knowledge that we accumulate in Chigen is not limited to cognitive domains, as explained in the previous sections. All human faculties participate in our experience, and Chigen grows through all of them. For instance, the knowledge associated with conviction—that is, the knowledge that moves us to action—is likewise born in Chigen. We may say that Chigen is all the knowledge imprinted or stored in a person's body, feelings, and spirit, and at the same time that personal knowledge with refined subjectivity controls all the functions of Chigen.

When we go beyond the limits of ordinary instruction to reach a student who seems hopeless, the result may be a special peaceful feeling of love toward the student, and we may feel encouraged to make a similar attempt with other students. Then later we may feel guilt for the incidents in which we neglected the needs of some other students, and we may commit ourselves not to repeat those mistakes. How do we define this feeling? If spiritual science advances, we may understand it much better, but we cannot fully articulate it now, yet it may be decisive in creating a general change in our attitude.

Since practice engages almost all the faculties of personhood, it is very likely that in the course of practice we are inspired and our eyes are opened. "I come to some answers every time I teach a course . . . learning is not school—learning is life," say Baskett and Hill (1990, 35). I have a habit of walking around or doing a simple chore when I become stuck while solving difficult problems. Many solutions occur to me while my body is engaged in something other than just sitting and thinking, one of many mysterious connections in the network of our knowledge base.

An important aspect of Chigen is the attitude we cultivate towards the unknown, which will greatly affect our ability to acquire the greatest benefit from our practice. The knowledge we obtain in practice is contextual. We often need to retain our knowledge of a crude reality, including as much of its context as possible, since we do not know when such knowledge may be useful. Frequently an apparently irrelevant or meaningless piece of knowledge becomes very significant later in an unanticipated situation. Thus, descriptions and interpretations are crucial elements of human actions (Zuber-Skerritt 1992, 78). By describing what we do, we can retain better what we learn, which is one of the reasons that description is so important in action research. We describe, retain, interpret, and reinterpret in order to enrich our local knowledge.

Conclusions

While the theories of action research promote respect for the agency and integrity of human beings, individual practitioners must be the ones to incorporate that respect into their work. Action research itself does not automatically guarantee the kind of attention and care that people need. It only provides the space for it.

At this point a question posed earlier becomes relevant: "Do we dare to ask our education system to allow practitioners and students a more complete exercise of their free agency?" The relationship that is implied by this question represents the inverse of reality. Action research should serve the improvement of education. But sometimes even an inappropriate question can shed light on an issue. If action research is sensitive to agency issues, it may help us in gauging to what extent we have fostered agency among practitioners.

I believe the actual effect of action research would be much greater if we are more aware of and more sensitive to agency issues. Action research provides a non-threatening environment in which practitioners can experiment in the exercise of their agency. Since action research is agency sensitive, action researchers become more aware of agency and learn to exercise their own agency, which prepares them to foster the agency of others. These are worthy efforts, whatever the cost. In my opinion, the ultimate goal of education—its crucial priority—is to assist personal growth and not to merely provide knowledge or development skills. Everything else is secondary to this growth, since the personal growth of individuals is the only true foundation of a lasting society.

The changes that result from action research, contrasted with those of the traditional sciences, are likely to be drastic, topological, and qualitative, rather than gradual, algebraic, and quantitative. Action research often changes the direction of a whole practice. Action research creates a new context for practice. Action research changes the attitudes of the practitioner.

The focal-subsidiary dichotomy in awareness generally dictates the limits of experiential learning. Because we cannot focus on more than one point at a time, innumerable factors escape our attention in our practice. Reflection (in the broadest sense of the term), which we will discuss in Chapter Five, is the key to overcoming this limitation.

Questions & Activities for Better Understanding

The following questions and suggestions are intended to stimulate further thinking. It may not be productive to follow them in a rigid manner. The readers are encouraged to modify questions/suggestions or create new questions/suggestions so that they can engage in truly meaningful thinking and learning.

1. Reflect on two similar situations at two different times in your practice (as practice you can choose any endeavor that is personally meaningful to you; e.g., your studies, career, interests, and so forth). Why are they different? What factors cause the two situations to be different? Try to predict and write down the outcomes of the next activity that you will do in your practice. After that activity, compare your prediction with the real outcomes. What are the recursive or stable elements in your practice and which are more volatile?

2. Search for any idea to improve your practice from your friends, experts, books, and so forth. Imagine the process where you implement that idea in your practice. Identify the issues that do not allow you to directly apply that idea to your practice. If possible, try that idea in your practice and see what positive outcomes as well as difficulties you come cross. If someone is available to collaborate with or assist you, share the outcomes with that person so that you can get feedback.

3. Pick out any activity in your practice that you recently did. Describe that activity as a sequence of different feelings that you experienced in the activity. If you were a robot without any feeling, how might have the outcomes of that activity been different? Identify the instances in which your feelings hamper or enhance the activity.

4. How do you respond to the idea of action research as a moral science? Do you trust the account of an action research while you know that the action researcher is dishonest? How can we build a trustworthy relationship among action research collaborators? Do we sometimes deceive ourselves? How can we tell whether or not we are whole-heartedly doing action research or not? What is the value of action research while our real motivation is not there?

5. Choose any activity in your practice. Select a 10-second to 1-minute segment of that activity and analyze what kinds of information are created in that activity segment. First, do it from your own perspective as a practitioner. Then, do it in your imagination as from an observer's perspective. Categorize those pieces of information that you obtained into two groups: articulated knowledge and tacit knowledge.

Chapter Four

Growing through Dialectic Process

Does a single cycle of action research overcome the gap between theory and practice? It rarely occurs with such ease. Usually the problems are solved through iterative adjusting and readjusting one's approach to the local reality. This chapter will investigate the power of dialectical process.

Because the process of practice is dialectical, a discussion of dialectical process might have properly been included in the preceding chapter, but it is such a copious subject with so many ramifications in action research that it deserves a chapter of its own. Among the many characteristics of the learning process that occur in practice, dialectical process is particularly important. It is a fundamental principle of progress in any practice; it is especially prominent in experiential learning.

Several descriptive terms that occur frequently in the literature on action research—i. e., *reflective, recursive, cyclic, spiral, dialogical,* and *dialectical*—are similar in meaning and are often used interchangeably; all of them refer to the same dialectical quality that characterizes the developmental process of practice. Many theorists use cyclic or spiral models to describe action research. Such a universal awareness of this concept underscores how essential dialectical process is to action research. Then how does this process occur in action research? During and after the events of our practice we may reflect on our performances. The results of reflection are continuously transformed into practice, and practice continuously generates reasons for reflection and development of these practical theories (Altrichter et al., 1991, 208).

The endless and ever-changing nature of both locality and practice, developed in previous chapters, indicates and calls for dialectical process, and contrasts with the static end of linear experimental process in the traditional sciences (Quigley 1995, 65). Here is the genius that can cope with the perpetual transformation of practice that is destined to outmode any potent general remedy or solution.

The navigational method mentioned in Chapter Three is well suited to explain the dialectic nature of action research. Since the circumstances of our practice are never fully anticipated and are continuously transient around us, we first move to the closest target in the direction that seems right based on the knowledge at hand (Suchman 1987, ix). We may not have abundant knowledge initially, but by reflecting on what we have accomplished and adjusting our course, we move on to the next target with new understanding and new knowledge. In this way, we advance closer and closer to the desired destination.

We use what we have in Chigen as a tentative scaffold from which to move on by stages. Observation, perception and description all depend on our understanding and interpretation, on the contents of Chigen, and then such contents depend upon that perception, observation, and description. Since Chigen is ever changing, the experiential knowledge accumulated in Chigen is always largely tentative. The eventual course of our practice gradually becomes known only as the nature of increasing factors bearing on our work unfolds to us. As one author puts it, we cannot tell what questions to ask until we observe the relevant phenomena closely and systematically (Wells 1994, 29). A grand plan at the beginning is, therefore, not practical, even though we need not give it up as we discussed before.

Without a constantly fine-tuned revision process, we will easily deviate from the most meaningful course of progress. Intensionality (the chief element of our action) necessarily involves ongoing reflexive monitoring of conduct (Manicas & Secord 1983, 408). Without this self-monitoring through reflection, we cannot truly own our practice. Because influences from a variety of sources may impinge upon our work, we must continually exert our agency to remain on a course that is in line with our intentions. The dialectical process that has been described so far can be summarized in a formula:

Practice + Chigen + Dialectical Process = Continual Progress

Thought and action (theory and practice) are dialectically related and should be understood as mutually constitutive (Pedretti & Hodson 1995, 469). This dialectic, or the relationship of theory and practice, is called "praxis." Praxis has to do with informed action which, when accompanied by reflection on its character and consequences, reflexively changes the "knowledge-base" which informs it (Carr & Kemmis 1986, 33). Thus, there is a dialectical relationship between theory arising from practice and practice improved by theory. In praxis, human beings are neither totally free subjects nor passive agents. They are producers and products of social reality (Zuber-Skerritt 1992, 27).

We overcome some of negative aspects of our biases through dialectic interaction. Our preconceptions, knowledge, skills, and all our faculties are tested and can be improved through direct contact with the reality of practice. Thus thought and action reinforce, benefit, and contribute to each other. We may speak of "togetherness" and "complementarity" of these partnered elements. Such a relationship is familiar in any human experience, which is periodically punctuated by the end of time units such as coffee break, day, week, month, season, year, and so forth. Thinking becomes action, and action becomes a never-ending cycle of re-creation (McNiff 1988, 51). And human beings are by nature reflexive individuals, generating and testing their hypotheses and applying them by way of example to their consciously controlled actions (Zuber-Skerrit, 1992). Although in larger scales, such as a group setting, people may consciously hypothesize and theorize important matters in their community for the betterment of their lives, common practitioners may not pay enough attention to the inner workings of their practice to intentionally formulate ideas and examine their assumptions. However, it is always true that every able practitioner is constantly monitoring his or her assumptions through acting in practice.

The process is also addressed from the perspective of increasing details. "Action research begins with a vague question which is only gradually clarified," (Zuber-Skerritt 1993, 55). Once action research begins, it continues as an iterative process. The results of reflection are continuously transformed into practice, and practice continuously generates reasons for reflection and development of these practical theories (Newby 1997, 80). Theories (and the ideas derived from theories) enlarge our vision by directing our attention to important aspects that would otherwise go unnoticed and by providing alternative frames for reinterpreting our experiences (Stevenson 1995, 201). Through this reciprocal course, the hazy question branches off in many directions, each of which leads us to a more delineated and lucid picture of that portion. As the traveler's metaphor in Chapter Two, as he or she closes in on the ancient mound (the target of interest), the more detail is revealed to him or her.

These descriptions above overlook some important points, however. When we frame praxis in terms of the interaction between action and Chigen, we can obtain a more complete picture of the process. As noted earlier, all of our faculties, not just the cognitive, are involved in growth and learning. Not only are thinking and theories a part of the dialectic of action, but other components are as well, such as feelings, tacit memory, and physical and spiritual functions. Any of innumerable such qualities may promote or impede and otherwise interplay significantly with action, so we discover that the words "thinking" and "theory" are not sufficiently inclusive. All the tacit elements in Chigen that strongly interact with action are also left out if we limit ourselves to the notions of thought or theory only.

An additional kind of complementarity exists in practice. The meaning of the part is determined by the meaning of the whole, while the knowledge of the whole is enriched by the knowledge of the parts (Wildemeersch 1992, 48). How can we implement this reciprocity? Fortunately, action research has a built-in mechanism to switch our mode of knowing from time to time. The Plan-Act-Evaluation cycle that we institute in an action research facilitates this mode shift. When we plan, holistic dioramas present backdrops against which we can layout our tactics. In action our foci stay with specific details of each part, which produces a new flow of information as we undergo the intact experiences of each action. Then, evaluation goes over the produced knowledge pieces to measure the progress in action by referencing to the whole scope. Thus, we can alternate our attention between the whole and the part as long as we initiate the action research cycle.

Why is planning so crucial in action research? Although it is extremely difficult to predict the consequences of an action, an attempt at prediction is sometimes essential to successful practice. We need to differentiate between what we can or should predict and what is impossible or inappropriate to predict, but it is aimless to plan without any expectation, and expectation naturally leads to prediction. Even in a extreme complexity, we need to do our best to estimate and predict so that we can plan appropriate action.

How does a plan enrich and refine Chigen? An old Asian saying, 温故知新 "On ko chi shin (By reviewing old things, we know new things)," reminds us of the importance to learn from the past. History is abounding with applicable lessons to our present and future. When we plan, we envision the future, and by recalling relevant experience from the past, we pre-evaluate things which might happen in the future. Thus we examine the contents of our Chigen to plan for future action. We mentally mark the things we feel are most essential for us to learn from practice. We also examine our feelings about possible future events. Our likes and dislikes help us to decide our future course. Motivation and ethical considerations may also be involved in planning.

As we have discussed, planning involves prediction, preview, pre-evaluation, pre-estimation, and so forth. The essence of a plan is activating and utilizing various elements in Chigen to meet the future needs of practice, including the improvement of the practice itself.

Lewin seems to have introduced the model of "a circle of planning, action, and fact-finding about the result of the action" (1946, 38). Later theorists have followed Lewin in using the circle (see Figure 1) as a model of the action research process. Deconstructing this model by a process similar to the one I used in the discussion of theory and practice, I began to feel that the model of a circle might be too mechanistic to apply to the procedures of action research. A circle seemed too simplistic, not organic enough to reflect the complex reality of practice. During planning stages we may do many fact-finding activities; action often requires revisions to a plan or new plans; fact-finding may occur at any stage of practice. Consequently, it seems that the idea of a set sequence, which a reader might infer from a circle, could be very misleading.

Likewise the term "plan" and "evaluation" seemed to me too heavy or technical to describe the very small steps that are sometimes associated with actions in practice, and I began to look for more general and inclusive words. But in the course of my reevaluation I became strongly convinced that these concepts are generally useful and that I cannot completely escape from the Lewin's diagram without losing significant elements of action research that affect successful improvement.

Nevertheless I want to present a dialectical model of my own as an alternative to Lewin's circle, as illustrated by two diagrams (see Figure 5-1 & 5-2). In Figure 1, the large circle represents the universe of an action research. The double pointed arrows denote dialectical process, which happens in all directions, in different magnitudes, and in different time extents. Probably, in reality, they are sometimes overlapping one another.

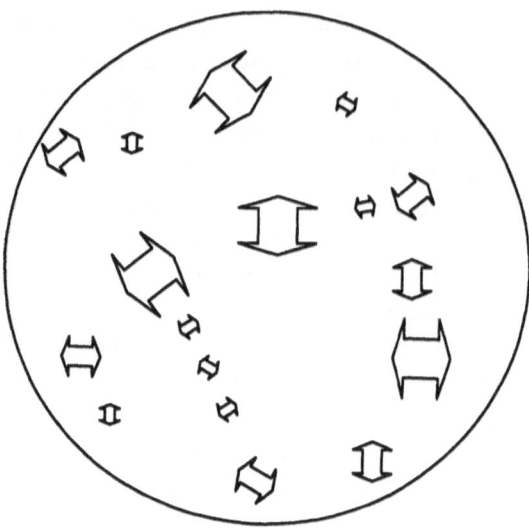

Figure 5-1

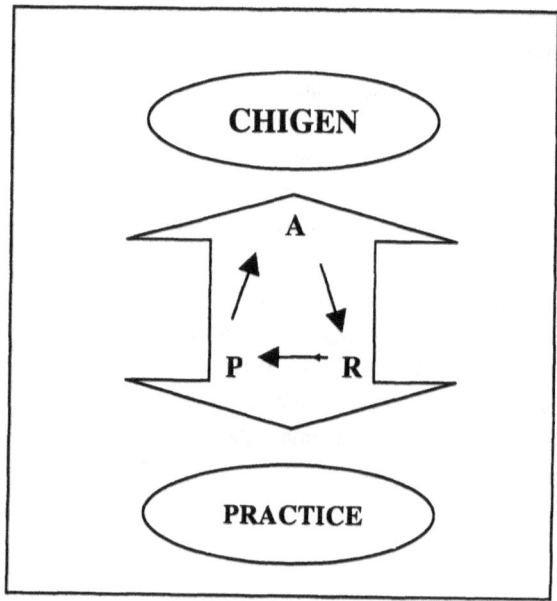

Figure 5-2

Figure 5-2 shows a close-up view of each arrow. The dialectical process is most comprehensively described as the interaction between Chigen and practice, which should incorporate cyclic procedures. Concerning the letters in the big arrow, P stands for preparation, A for action, and R for reflection. It is important to note that this cycle doesn't mean a single proceeding; it can and should repeat multiple times. In many contexts I prefer the terms "preparation" and "reflection" as they are less arcane and thus suitable to daily practice than Lewin's "plan" and "evaluation." My terms are more inclusive and more flexible as well. They meet the need I have noted previously to avoid the tendency to cover every possible contingency or detail as strictly as those technical terms may imply. There is a risk to waste precious resources on trivialities.

Preparation involves such elements as examining the justifications for actions, reflecting upon previous experiences, planning, and honing our faculties. Preparation may also include less obvious elements like play and pondering. The type of preparation will be dictated by the nature of the practice. Theoretically, preparation may take any number of forms. Sometimes our whole preparation may be the momentary thought before making up our mind. At other times a careful, more elaborate and collaborative preparation may be required. We take into account such components as the scale of the action, the time frame, availability of resources, degree of interest, and the priority we attach to the action.

Lewin describes the element of evaluation as "fact-finding about the result of the action" (1946, 38). "Fact-finding" is a better choice of words than "evaluation" in that the former sounds less technical or esoteric than the latter, yet it conveys the essential and practical meaning of this process to practitioners. Without this element, practice remains just one of many experiences that may pass by without leaving any significant trace of learning. By directing our attention to the facts generated in and about our practice, our experiential learning increases substantially. Sensible or reflective practitioners never fail to learn something from the facts they discover about their practice. That is one of the reasons I feel that the term "reflection" may be more suitable than "evaluation." But whatever we call it, we cannot improve our practice without this step.

The complementary interaction or dialectic between Chigen and practice is constant and never ending. They enhance each other. This dialectic has to be expanded to include preparation and reflection, which should also recur during the entire process of practice. In either preparation or reflection, we are not directly acting in practice. Outwardly, we are inactive and static. Is that seemingly dormant period justifiable in the midst of a demanding practice? The following example may give us new insight to look at this situation.

The Zen Buddhist phrase *"muga no kyouchi"* describes a state of mind which I have tried to approximate in English by "selflessness" or "void." Zen became one of the mental supports for the Japanese Samurai warriors, whose traditions and spirit are still alive in the high work ethic of present Japanese businessmen. A vital aspect of the spiritual training of the Samurai was *Za-zen* (sitting meditation). *Za-zen*, which unfortunately today's businessmen no longer practice, incorporates *"muga no kyouchi"* and is an apparently inactive, and in the physical sense absolutely unproductive, endeavor, involving motionless sitting and meditating. Its ultimate purpose is total enlightenment, but it is understood that even without achieving that goal, practitioners derive great benefit from obtaining even one new insight. Many beneficial insights are the usual experience. Paradoxically, this apparently inefficacious act can be the most productive time in a practitioner's life. In losing oneself, the true self is found. Applying to action research this Zen philosophy that nothingness can prove very fruitful reinforces the idea that reflection itself may produce more meaningful changes in practice than devoting oneself in an activity or just following the rigidly structured system of plan, action, and evaluation.

Any step we take in action research needs to provide stable ground for successive steps. This is the key to a successful dialectical process, and frequent reflection provides the basis for this smooth transition by balancing efforts, avoiding redundancy, introducing more effective ideas, and so forth..

Questions & Activities for Better Understanding

> The following questions and suggestions are intended to stimulate further thinking. It may not be productive to follow them in a rigid manner. The readers are encouraged to modify questions/suggestions or create new questions/suggestions so that they can engage in truly meaningful thinking and learning.

1. Why is repetition so important in action research? How does any general idea fail to work in an ever-changing local situation of a practice? What are the key steps of the cyclic process of action research? What may be the danger of rigidly following the prescribed action research cycle? List the factors that prevent a grand plan from working well especially at the beginning of the action research.

2. Why are the three elements (practice, Chigen, and dialectical process) in the formula for continuous progress essential? Can we succeed without the complete set of those elements? Consider the following example: One worker is dismayed by the poor compensation that he has received for the last ten years. He or she approaches the administrator and asks, "Why haven't you raised my salary for these years, while I have become an experienced worker through these accumulated years?" Then, the administrator responds, "Certainly, you have accumulated many years, but you have virtually repeated the same thing for ten times without improvement."

3. Any human experience is replete with repetitive activities. Why do many people fail to make the most of them? In what way can we identify recursive components in our activity or create spiral procedures to upgrade our performance? At the beginning of an action research, why is it often necessary to start with a vague plan and objective? What kind of attitude should we develop so that we can appropriately deal with such vagueness and uncertainty?

4. Why did the author introduce an alternative model of the action research dialectic that Figure 5-1 and 5-2 illustrate? What is a pitfall of the traditional model of a single cycle described in Figure 1? What are the significant points of the P-A-R cycle embedded in the big arrow of Figure 5-2? Why shouldn't we neglect the fact that we can repeat the cycle multiple times?

5. Do we habitually and systematically create an open space in our mind and schedule where we can do nothing else but ponder, in a positive way, on im-

portant issues associated with our increasingly demanding modern practice? Why can "muga no kyouchi" or the "state of selfless or void" be productive? How meaningful to ponder and meditate in the modes of preparation and reflection? How do these two modes facilitate pondering and meditation?

Chapter Five

Systematic Reflection

Reflection
Every time she looked in a mirror
She saw precisely what she expected
Until she went beyond the boundaries
To explore the crevices and peaks.

The layers of her reflection
Were not easily seen at first
They hid behind her perceptions
Laying dormant until she searched.
And long after her inviting—
Editing and coloring went on
Shading in an understanding
Of who she thought she was.

But many parts of equal importance
Got lost without her knowing
So now when she looks at her reflection
She tries to go beyond
To see what she cannot.
(Vullianm, 1992, 140-141)

We may consider practice an engine that propels action research to cross the gap and systematic reflection the steering wheel that guides action research to the most meaningful route to achieve its goal.

Because of its close connection with dialectical process, reflection (reflexivity) was discussed at some length in the previous chapter. This chapter treats systematic, as opposed to casual, reflection. The extra knowledge produced by systematic reflection makes the crucial difference between ordinary experiential learning and action research. However, it is not possible or necessary to clearly distinguish between the part of practice that is directly related to action research and the part that is not. Saying "the knowledge generated by the practice" is quite often equivalent to saying "the knowledge generated by the action research." Therefore, it is the degree of systematicity that distinguishes action research from experiential learning, which is naturally happening in practice.

Dictionaries define "reflection" as "deep and careful thought." Action research adds "extensive and organized" to "deep and careful." These supplemented dimensions can generate far more knowledge than does the ordinary reflection of experiential learning. As noted many times, practice heavily depends on our understanding and interpretation of reality. Reflection lays the basis of that ability to understand and interpret, and continuous reflection recreates and upgrades those abilities. Reflection occurs at all stages of action research. Reflection starts, advances, and completes planning, thus guiding the course of action. It initiates, promotes, and refines evaluation.

We speak of reflection, and also of meta-self-reflection, which is the reflection on each one of the faculties of personhood. We reflect on our self, feelings, physical abilities, and so forth.

Although many authors emphasize systematicity in action research (Kelly 1985; Stenhouse 1981; Manicas & Secord 1983; McCutheon & Jung 1990; Reason 1993; Elden & Chisholm 1993; Zuber-Skerritt 1992b; Wells 1994; Gianotti 1994), they do not seem to agree on the form that systematicity should take.

My own working definition of "systematicity" is doing whatever it takes, in as organized a way as possible, to obtain more data than usual, which is a base line. Action researchers can legitimately employ higher systematicity and are encouraged to do so whenever the situation allows them without hampering their practice. It is true that such a definition may be an oversimplification or even a contradiction to the usage of the traditional sciences, but it suits the approach of action research. The unpredictability of practice makes it almost impossible to decide in advance where and how to find the most important data and when to reflect on it. As quoted in a previous chapter, "One could never be too diligent about recording all aspects of the research process, for, over time, the seemingly insignificant becomes relevant" (Noffke 1995, 90). However, defining systematicity to restrict to rigorous predetermined procedures is not only impossible but also incongruous, because it may put unreasonable restrictions on the natural development of practice.

The first requirement of systematicity in action research is to obtain extra information from our practice, an idea that corresponds well with Lewin's notion of "fact-finding." The second requirement to be considered is organization. We organize our time and efforts so that we can obtain data regularly and frequently, from as many independent sources as possible, and reflect upon it. We do not have to collect data according to any external criteria except our own particular purpose. The practitioner decides where to focus and what kind of data to collect based on the needs of his or her practice. These two requirements, extra data collection and organization, are the core to define systematicity within action research. Some readers might be concerned with the quality of the information obtained by mere increase of data. Of course the quality of information is important. The quality-check of action research, however, doesn't always follow the rigid linear procedure of traditional sciences. The action research dialectics has its own built-in system to check the quality. In action research information is obtained first by organizing data gathering, second by carefully reflecting on the data, and finally by verifying the data through practice, though not necessarily in such a rigidly prescribed fashion. Repeatedly, every time we go through the cyclic process, the reality-check takes place, and that check in the practice is the best test to verify the quality of the information.

If we exclude systematicity from action research, we lose the important information that an ordinary practitioner's eyes cannot access, due to the distinction between focal and subsidiary awareness. We need a backup system to retain information that could otherwise escape our attention because the focal fixation prevents us from seeing it. Reviewing and pondering collected data that may have seemed unimportant can produce additional insight. Systematicity provides a reservoir by increasing both the quality and the quantity of information that we can obtain. The diversity of ideas generated by systematicity, when it facilitates growth in the practitioner, has a long-lasting effect on practice.

Clearly pre-specified procedures or prescriptions, if they do not derive from the research situations, may be more harmful than beneficial to action research. For this reason, specificity is not a part of the general definition of systematicity in action research, but grows out of the conditions of the particular action research. Organized fact-finding is a general requirement of action research, but specificity must be defined locally. The process presented in this chapter for building systematicity into research should be seen neither as prescriptive, nor as invariable, characteristics which would be contradictory to the spirit of action research, but rather as an essential supplementary source of ideas, tools, or opportunities.

In the traditional sciences the aim of systematicity is to obtain accurate, valid, and objective information about an object or phenomenon in order to see it clearly and eventually to control it. Systematicity is supposed to increase the validity of the knowledge that a study generates. In action research, however, we often want to obtain diverse information for a better understanding or interpretation of the target. For example, if we can only develop a different perspective that leads to an improvement of practice, or if through systematic reflection we acquire some encouraging facts that engender more enthusiasm for our practice, then systematicity is functioning at that pertinent junction of the action research. Therefore, the data can play new roles that help refine and enhance the subjective functions of the action researchers, thus enriching and elevating their Chi-gen in addition to its traditional roles. Another example is that descriptions of researchers' feelings are regarded as relevant and crucial in action research, while they are irrelevant and out of place in the traditional sciences. Thus, while the traditional sciences aim to control the target phenomena according to human wish by rigidly systematic research method which seeks convergence as a sign of validity, action research aspires to empower human agency to take its own course by providing divergent ideas. In order to support human development, the pertinent systematicy must be flexible or loosely standardized so that agency may maintain optimal control over its action.

Action research organizes data collection based on the unique needs and situations of the practice rather than against an external general, and often irrelevant standard. Nonetheless, there are some generic techniques that have been developed in other fields of study that can be adapted to action research. For instance, triangulation, the use of multiple independent data sources, is one of the techniques used in social sciences to validate the resultant information. If other independent researchers verify the notion obtained from a source of data, or if findings resulting from multiple observations converge to a certain conclusion, we can generally determine that such a notion or conclusion is trustworthy. Sometimes we may want to make sure that our decision making is based on reliable findings before actually applying them in practice. Yet, the validity of these findings is eventually tested in practice since the application process itself is the process of validation (for further discussion on validity, see Table 1 in Chapter Three). If the findings work, then they are acceptable; if they don't work, then they are useless or invalid. In any case, whenever possible, triangulation should be employed in action research. Quigley (1995, 64) confirms this point by saying that we may use "multiple investigators, multiple sources of data, or multiple methods to confirm the emerging findings...[in other words, we may use] 'pooled judgment'" to increase validity. McKernan (1991, 23) also supports this point. When findings from triangulation converge, it is a good sign for high reliability and validity. It is vital to reiterate an important point here. The on-going discussion does not mean that action research should stay with primitive, casual, or easy-to-use data collection techniques. Whenever the timing is proper, we can employ any rigorous and elaborate technique to glean scrupulous and unbiased information. The point is that any technique should not be imposed externally unless significant positive long-term effects are expected by doing so, but principally the local conditions should dictate the choice.

In reality, divergence may be the more common result of triangulation, and in action research this does not nullify the research findings, as we discussed above. Diversity is not necessarily a weakness of the systematicity in action research as long as such discoveries lead to sundry perspectives, deeper understanding, and eventually an advanced practice. Logical leaps are common in practice as well as in reflection. Any idea that is intuitively derived from any observation, thought, idea, theory or perspective without scrutinizing the logical sensibility of its incipient process can be significant and productive in action research.

On the other hand, the traditional view of validity seems to have more relevance to action research than some action research theorists are willing to acknowledge (see Walace, 1987, 107; Altrichter et al. 1993, 155; and Corey 1953). Although validity does not occupy the supreme position in action research that it does in the traditional sciences, the priority is nevertheless high enough to secure and improve the minimum validity of action research. Improvement must be based on truth no matter what it may be objective or subjective, and the standards of validity are still important tools in determining what the truth is.

There are a few additional ways to look at this issue. The validity that action research is concerned with depends on particular practice situation, which implies that the validity of a certain piece of knowledge is measured by the generalizability or transferability of that knowledge to a particular situation. One way to generalize or transfer findings from one situation to another is "naturalistic generalization, arrived at by recognizing the similarities of objects and issues in and out of context and by sensing the natural covariations and happenings. To generalize this way is to be both intuitive and empirical" (Stake 1980, 68-69). McKernan (1991, 4) writes of validating through practice as we discussed above, and Sharples (1983) sees validity in terms of authenticity and accountability. Although we desire a minimum level of practical accuracy, we do not require absolute accuracy or broadly generalizable trustworthiness for the knowledge of action research to be valid.

Articulation, robustness, and rigor relate closely to validity. These concepts are often considered the aim of systematicity by the traditional sciences. But while they have their place in action research, we assign them less importance than the traditional sciences do. The crucial point here is balance. Argyris and Schön say, "the challenge is to define and meet standards of appropriate rigor without sacrificing relevance" (1991, 85). Finding this balance is indeed a challenge, for as the previous discussions have suggested, when we inflict methodological rigor in action research, we may impede the natural progress of practice. Often we must first sacrifice rigor, then later, when we are less constrained by the situation, we can back up and restore the quality of examination, which has been less than ideal due to the lost rigor. In certain favorable situations, we may be able to make a careful plan in which we can join rigor with relevance. Only rarely is it necessary to put rigor first because the potential gain cannot override the loss of relevance, which may evoke unredeemable aftermath. Therefore, we must always be keenly aware that the purpose of action research is to serve the practice, and not vice versa.

Systematicity in the traditional sciences is synonymous with objectification, and the traditional sciences try to exclude all subjective judgments. But in action research, idiosyncrasy and bias are not always categorically undesirable; it depends on the context. Sometimes we must modify or discard our biases to accord with the more universal perspective that opens up to us in our research. Biases can at times hinder our personal development as well as render our practice ineffective. But some personal peculiarities are harmonious with our practice and supportive of it, and we want to keep them as the personal signatures we place on practice. For example, if you favor Method X over Method Y—the former simply fits your style and thus works better—despite the statistical fact that more people are successful with Method Y in a comparable situation, you may be better off with your favorite method. The systematicity of action research, however, allows us to somewhat objectively examine our knowledge base whenever the timing is congruous, thus makes us less vulnerable to potentially harmful biases.

"By distancing ourselves from the flow of activities, we have a better chance of dealing with the problems that entangle us; redefining them and reorganizing our response" (Altrichter et al. 1993, 206). Distancing is not the same as completely removing ourselves, though, and we can be organized or systematic while simultaneously valuing subjectivity.

Occasionally practitioners may need to present data in a way that is acceptable to the traditional scientists, which requires a different order of systematicity to meet the standard of credibility and authenticity of that particular audience. However, the more rigorous systematicity we impose upon our practice, the more restricted our practice will be. There are great benefits in such a rigorously systematic approach, but these benefits do not come without cost. It is therefore necessary to find the level of systematicity that will serve our practice best. Progress in research is optimized by examining high-priority problems, looking for the meaning in them, and framing probing questions that have not yet been articulated in those particular problems, rather than by looking for solutions to theoretical problems selected by someone else.

We may define science as any systematic study of our reality through which we can better describe, articulate, and understand reality and thus improve our life. Although action research has a quite different set of methodologies from the traditional sciences, it fits perfectly our definition of science. The difference lies in the nature of systematicity. The traditional scientists may criticize action research for its lack of precision in articulating phenomena, but the traditional sciences cannot shed as much light on human behavior at locality. Although articulation in action research may be somewhat fuzzy and incomplete especially at the beginning, significant and essential knowledge can originate from such attempts.

In summary, the ultimate purpose of systematicity in action research is specifically assisting the subjectivity of a particular individual to develop and be relined instead of striving after more rigorous objectivity, which rather serves for a general purpose that may not be highly relevant to the local situation. The key to successfully maintaining the systematicity of action research lies in mindfully balancing between rigor and relevance. How can we manage this challenging task? We will now turn our attention to the fact that the whole action research process occurs through the medium of reflection so that we may recognize that a decisive role reflection can take in maneuvering this delicate balancing task.

Reflection is possible and important at all stages of research. Altrichter and others explain, "In teachers' action research, there is no separation between stages of knowledge construction (reflection) and testing (action). Reflection takes place partly in action, and even reflection-on-action is not limited to particular research stages" (1993, 209). We reflect on all aspects of practice. This is the universality of reflection.

Another quality of reflection is its organic character. Through reflection we may obtain a beautiful theory, realization or enlightenment. The result may be very clear, well organized, and simple, even when the process of reflection itself may be inarticulate and even frustrating and arduous. We often explain the functions of reflection by an articulate model partly because its product, the knowledge that we are aware of, is articulate, while the real reflective process is clandestine. An analogy might clarify this point. A pearl is a simple and beautiful gem. However, both the pearl-making process and the producer, the oyster, are complex and, from one point of view, ugly. They, nevertheless, serve superbly as the bridge between the pearl and the world.

The functions of reflection are far more complex than a single model can describe. We have little knowledge of how ideas are produced in reflection or how reflection influences actions. The depth of the relationships between reflection and our faculties is far beyond our comprehension. However, it is very clear that all of these elements are interactively engaged in the process of reflection.

A brief glimpse at the inner workings of reflection may be apropos here. As discussed in Chapter Three, feelings play a much greater role in action research than may be obvious at first. Feelings evoke, carry out, sustain, change the course of, and terminate reflection. But at the same time reflection evokes, carries out, sustains, changes the course of, and terminates feelings. Reflection and feelings are mutually dependent and interactive on a deep level. Another indispensable point is that reflection observes and monitors feelings, and this relationship is not reversible. How is it possible for this relation to be so enigmatic? One principal answer lies in focal and subsidiary awareness. Anxiety may keep our focus on the problematic point as we reflect for solutions. Once we turn our focus in reflection from the agitating issue, the emotions will subside. I on another instance, an unforeseen issue causes strong feelings; then these feelings grab attention (focus) and consequently ignite reflection on that issue as well. Once the concern is resolved in reflection, the feelings recede and the focus moves on to another issue. The relationships are not just with feelings; reflection is intricately related with every aspect of Chigen.

Chapter Two described how the double awareness (focal and subsidiary) generates uniqueness and limitations in our knowledge acquisition. Reflection follows the same principles. At any moment in reflection we can direct our focus to any given point in either the theoretical or real world. This fact gives us boundless freedom, and we can shape our reflection according to our personal choice. Reflection is very personal. One can create a space in reflection with perfect freedom from the outside world. Thus external factors cannot completely compel reflection in any particular way about any given topic. Agency is absolute in this decision. The only constraint on the course of reflection is the moral standard in each of us. In this sense, action research depends on our ethics.

We are limited in that we can direct our focus mainly to one point at a time, both an advantage and a disadvantage. Since we can process only a limited amount of information simultaneously, it is to our advantage to have one source of information at a time so that we are not overwhelmed. The consequence of this is that we cannot reflect on things that are in a subsidiary awareness, which is why collecting information for more than immediate needs is considered as the first requirement or premise of systematicity.

The role of reflection in Chigen is divided into three dimensions. First, reflection generates meaning, understanding, and interpretations of phenomena, which refines and organizes Chigen so that it may produce intelligent judgment. At the same time subjectivity is refined and upgraded. Second, reflection organizes, directs, and monitors the process of planning, action, and evaluation, which enriches Chigen with procedural information. Third, reflection observes and monitors each one of our faculties (meta-faculty information), which prepares Chigen to produce intelligent actions by keeping equilibrium among the faculties.

Although Elden and Chrisholm (1993, 127) start with John Dewey's belief that intellectual inquiry begins with a problematic situation, we can broaden the condition for inquiry beyond Dewey's meaning. Our inquiry should start wherever we have interest, desire, motivation, goal, purpose, vision, hope, ethical obligation, and so forth. Our inquiry applies not only to an immediate problem, but also to our overall pursuit for a better and more moral existence. Wise ethical judgments are the basis of good intelligent practice, which, in turn, sustains our society. They are also the basis of action research.

In order to create a true science from action research, we must not only develop appropriate ways to organize data collection and reflection, and establish suitable methodologies and epistemologies, but we must also acknowledge the proper position of morality, the spiritual dimension, as an indispensable base of the science. Without honesty how can we trust the data? How can we entrust our private data to a person with unethical intentions? How can we succeed in our endeavors with people if we are horribly self-centered?

Even though we can not fully grasp the operation of reflection in its entirety, we know empirically that there are certain activities that lead to more fulfilling reflection. Reflection becomes significantly careful and meaningful when we enter the modes of *recording*, *reviewing*, and *reporting*, which lift reflection from the ground of experiential learning to the level of science. Each of them is a necessary aspect of reflection in action research. Without them, reflection remains crude, volatile, casual, and susceptible to misconception.

Recording is any effort to maintain data involved with the practice. Data may be contained in a journal or a log, on an audio or video recording, or in a photograph, drawing, portfolio, scrapbook, questionnaire, official document, letter, email, and so forth. Methods of data collection are not constrained in any particular way. There is no limit to the material that may be classified as data, as long as it is related to the practice and can be used as a reference to any overlooked or forgotten aspect of our experience when we reflect upon it in the future.

Once information leaves the practitioner's mind or is culled from other sources to be stored, it begins to function in a variety of unpredictable ways. Its uses are unlimited. It benefits not only the practitioner himself or herself but also others. Once the data is published or otherwise made available to the public, further investigation becomes possible for others.

Recording gives names to the undefined and sheds light on nebulous ideas in Chigen and experience. Through this process of articulation we begin to see phenomena more clearly, and we perceive many hidden details. Recording enables us to monitor our reactions and better interpret reality. There are many other interesting fruits of this mode of reflection. (See the "writing to learn" movement, e. g., Zinsser, 1988.)

Recording also provides a beneficial detachment of the information from the practice and from the practitioner. The data take on a life of their own; setting off information that was not available before reflection. Recording provides not only a store of information but also many other benefits, such as the articulation of thought, the consequent discovery of hidden premises, the attainment of detached or objective knowledge about the experience that, in practice, completely engages our attention and so forth.

In collecting data we start with the points we are interested in as a practitioner. Since we cannot know which data will be meaningful in the later stage of action research, we must collect as much extra data as our circumstances allow. It is important not to neglect recording our feelings and our observations of our other faculties. Since the major part of the experiential learning related to these faculties is tacit and, therefore, too evasive to reflect on effectively, the data must supply pointers that mark and elucidate tacit elements. Additionally, as we discussed the three dimensions in which refection assists Chigen to grow, we should include these three dimensions: the versatile and in-depth interpretation of our experience, the orchestration and management of action research cycle, and the monitoring of all our faculties in the process of a bpractice.

Recording is necessary because our capacity to absorb or process information is limited, and we therefore need to store what we are not presently focused on for later reflection. We need verbalized knowledge to organize and lead our reflection, since verbalized or articulate knowledge is the matrix of the reasoning and logical thinking which constitute the backbone of reflection. The verbalized portion of knowledge accumulated in recording and the non-verbal knowledge to which they may direct our attention help us reconstruct in our mind the phenomena that we reflect upon in action research.

A Japanese translation of a teaching of Confucius (551-479 B. C.), 思いて学ば ざれば即ち暗く学びて思わざれば即ち危うし (Omoite manabazareba sunawachi kuraku, manabite omowazareba sunawachi ayaushi may be rendered in English as "Our life remains unenlightened if we think without learning, but it becomes dangerous if we learn without thinking." This proverb may serve to introduce the discussion of *reviewing*. Reviewing is a process in which we turn our focal awareness to our record. We cannot reflect in a vacuum. Memory often fails to recall needed information, as memory storage gradually fades. The review process feeds our mind with data for reflection. We can subdivide the materials to review into three groups. We review our own record, we review feedback from others concerning our findings, and we review additional materials, especially related literature.

In reviewing our own record we reflect on the reality we reconstruct from that record. Each time we review, we reconstruct reality, and every time we do so somewhat differently. A new situation induces us to interpret the record in a particular way, which yields additional understanding about the practice in question. The same record may be reviewed many times, finding new meaning each time. The insignificant becomes significant. We cannot review without reflecting. In this mode, reflection becomes, again, careful and meaningful.

In reviewing others' feedback our subjectivity can be examined and refined by ways of thinking other than our own. We can look at our practice from different angles. Since our location limits what we see, we naturally develop particular and idiosyncratic perspectives, which may still be crude, undeveloped, and therefore ineffective to deal with even a particular local case. Others' view can complement, enrich, and refine our view, so that we can better understand, handle, and improve the local situations of practice. It is also through interacting with others that we realize our own distinct identity. In this review process, reflection refines our subjectivity and synchronically defines our uniqueness.

Reviewing related literature guides us to more secure paths in our practice. "A little knowledge is dangerous" because, being often fragmented and lacking sufficient context, it leads easily to erroneous courses. We should collect as much information, in literature, related to our practice as possible so as to have a comprehensive picture of what we are engaging in, and thus to increase our likelihood of making sound decisions. Both general studies and case studies in the same or related field offer special insights into our own practice.

Reporting is any means of communication through which we share with others the knowledge that we learn from our action research. It includes any dialogue that we have with our colleagues and associates concerning our findings and any form of publication of those findings. When we think about an audience in speaking or writing, we reorganize our knowledge to meet the needs of that audience. This is a very interesting phenomenon and is another excellent arena for reflection. Although Stenhouse (1975) insists that researchers must publish their findings and that we cannot call an endeavor "research" without reporting it, for many practitioners, publication is almost impossible, and even discussing their findings may be impossible or prohibited in their situation. Therefore, we must be careful in judging whether or not we should include this mode in order to call our endeavor action research. Although this mode definitely gives meaningful dimension for reflection, a facilitator should not discourage those who cannot formally share their findings with others to conduct action research. On the other hand, they should be advised to write some form of summary that is supposed to address other than themselves, even when such a summary may not be shared immediately. Such a record can serve as another source for reviewing.

Summary

This chapter has defined meaningful reflection of action research in two ways. First, reflection must be based on a more grounded knowledge base than experiential learning. And such knowledge base is constantly updated by systematic fact-finding. Second, the true power of reflection is manifest in its three major modes: recording, reviewing, and reporting. Reflection works to refine our Chigen and thus all of our faculties, which reside in Chigen. Chigen is both the knowledge base and the power source for practice. Chigen is not enhanced easily just by reading, or by listening to lectures, or by other forms of passive learning. It requires dynamic interaction between the whole person and the reality of practice. It also requires meaningful reflection. Planning (Preparation), action, and evaluation (fact-finding & reflection) are the most fruitful and meaningful steps for Chigen to grow or develop. These three steps are embedded in reflection, which monitors, organizes, and leads them, and which is most effective and productive when all three of the modes are employed.

Questions & Activities for Better Understanding

The following questions and suggestions are intended to stimulate further thinking. It may not be productive to follow them in a rigid manner. The readers are encouraged to modify questions/suggestions or create new questions/suggestions so that they can engage in truly meaningful thinking and learning.

1. What is the difference between the experiential learning that naturally happens in practice and action research? What two requirements characterize the systematicity that action research employs in data gathering and reflection? Why is it not productive to impose pre-specified system on action research procedure? When are more rigid systems appropriate in action research?

2. Why is the mere increment of data so significant in action research? How is this point explained by the two awareness distinctions? If the research results are divergent, does this mean that such results are not valid in action research? How does action research look at such divergence? What kind of data are you interested in gathering for your action research? How do you initially collect data? What is your expectation about the evolution process of your data collection method?

3. Consider a weeklong experiment of data collection. The following steps may give you meaningful and eye-opening, hand-on experiences:
   (a) Imagine what kind of knowledge and experience this data collection may generate. Write down major points from your imagination for future reference.
   (b) How do you like to organize your data collection? Where, when, how, how often, and by who do you keep record of your performance in practice?
   (c) Implement your plan in your action research.
   (d) After that week, reflect on the data and write down what you have learned from that one-week experience and reflection.
   (e) Compare the data from Step (a) with the data from Step (d). Identify those points that you could imagine happening and those points that you would never expect to happen. Why are the latter points difficult to predict?

4. What are the guiding principles that help us decide the balance between rigor and relevance when we consider the level of systematicity? What are

the three dimensions of the reflection's contributions to Chigen? How do these dimensions inform us of the areas where we can search for meaningful data?

5. Why does reflection become more meaningful and productive in the three modes (recording, reviewing, and reporting)? How can we carefully reflect if we do not employ any of these three modes? The following activities may help you recognize the power of refection.

    a. During or after one day's practice, record your activities for a certain period of time (e.g., 30 minutes). A few days later review what you recorded. Discuss that experience either in your log or with your associates.

    b. Visit a near-by library and consult with a reference librarian to find relevant literature that may provide you with ideas to improve your practice. After reading the related literature for a few hours, reflect on and write about the thoughts that occurred during the reading.

Chapter Six

Lived Experience of Action Research: Five Evolving Case Studies

The previous five chapters discussed the general or universal natures of those five essential principles of action research. In this chapter my personal or local episodes are utilized in the hopes of enriching the readers' understanding about the action research experience from the aspect of application. I will reflect below on the five cases (tutoring, fatherhood, a family game, facilitation of a student's implementation, and professional performance) that changed the view and performance of my personal and professional life; some are not typical topics on which action research is commonly employed. Thus, I will prove how extensively, in our personal path, we can apply action research to cultivate any facet of our life as well as illustrate how the five principles made action research experiences meaningful and empowering, and identify major impacts of these experiences on my personal and professional growth.

The purpose of this chapter is not to explicate each case in such details that the readers can replicate the same or similar experience. Knowing from the previous chapter's discussion that rich description of an experience can breed naturalistic generalization, I would like to keep each description terse and turn the focus onto the major episodes so that they may more effectively delineate the essential nature of action research experience. I believe that the readers are ready to embark their own quest and I should no burden them with excessive description. However, it may be appropriate to add some notes here to my general action research procedure and record keeping system, even though they are doubtlessly the products of my peculiar personal indulgence.

During the last ten years I attempted dozens of small and large action research projects. Some were very brief and casual and a few were longitudinal like the fifth case study. The majority was my solo projects and just a few were collaborative ones. Some were just ideas; after writing down the plans they did not go anywhere. After ten years' experience, I feel that action research is an essential part of my life, which is constantly molding my Chigen with many unexpected findings. It is often difficult to clearly distinguish the action research part of my life from the rest because they are merged in a very intricate way.

Although my recording system is constantly evolving, the basic organization became somewhat stable after a couple of years' experience. My basic recording device is extremely low-tech or no-tech and inexpensive: pen, letter-size paper, and folder. I often use the backside of a printed sheet (I majored in forestry!). Occasionally I use audio and video recording. Computers are usually used when I need to create formal documents. Every year I produce about one thousand page in a general log which records everything including my personal information concerning family events, finance, shopping, church affairs, friends, health, and so forth. However, the majority of these records are directly related to various action research projects. The filed sheets are eventually three-hole punched and kept in a binder. The ten years' record takes about four to five-foot-wide space on the bookshelf.

There are three major ideas in my recording that seem to make it more productive. Everything is kept in chronological order. I keep the flow of thinking/writing running as smoothly as possible and keep enough margins in each page for later entries. I will expand these points a little further.

1. If we cannot retrieve an important piece of information effectively, the record is worthless. Therefore, I must make each sheet distinct and each important passage stand out. Each sheet has the date/page information on the top-right corner. If today is July 14th 2007 and I am writing the 8th page on that day, the identification number for that page may look

like 07/14/07-8. This numbering-system works well for me because I sometimes misplace some sheets from the record and they are left there for months. At other occasions when I am working on the issue that ranges over many different time periods, the sheets from different files might get mixed up one another. Since we can scarcely finish our task in one sitting, there is always such a risk. Color-highlighting and colored sticky notes that are visible from outside of the file are effective for faster information retrieval.

2. I know some associates who seem to be able to directly write down ideas in a way that others can easily follow. But I tend to jot down everything that comes into mind and that I feel important enough for future reference. Oftentimes, when stuck in thinking, I raise questions in writing, and then those questions propel and rubricate further thinking. So the end results of writing can be quite fragmented, inconsistent, illogical, or confusing for others; in fact they can be so even for myself when I review them later. Therefore, when I read the uncertain passages at a later time, I insert a dated comment to clarify the points. Such a procedure is important to me for two reasons. First, since our recording time is usually very restricted, we must optimize it by fully engaging our mind in thinking and writing. For that purpose, I keep the natural flow of thoughts in writing and let the recording system revise and refine the record through continuous reviewing and rewriting cycle. Second, the free-flow of thinking leads to new ideas and awareness. We humans seem to be unable to see what may lie in our future thinking. Talking about predicting outcomes of our thinking, we are, so to speak, 'surrounded by the thick mist of darkness.' Beyond one moment's thought is murkiness. Therefore, by letting our thought take its own course, we are led to astoundingly unexpected ideas.

3. It is wise not to fill out each page. First, it is burdensome to read through crammed letters. Second, additional ideas quite often occur to us after we scribble ideas. Therefore, leaving wide margins is a good investment. While writing, at times our intuition signals that some passages are worthy of further contemplation. Usually I underline two types of sentences: good questions and synopses of organized thought (e.g., hypothesis, belief, principle, etc.) that I number according to the order of appearance on the same page (Q1, Q2, ...for questions and *1, *2, ...for synopses). If I refer to a specific underlined sentence, the reference number looks like 07/17/07-8-*1, which corresponds to the sen-

tence that appears on the 8th page of July 17th, 2007. Among some synopses, that particular one is the number one on that page.

Tutoring

This pilot study was a very simple case study. There were two parts: three 30-45 minutes tutoring sessions with my son and several one-hour sessions with a male junior high student, for which sessions I was paid. Each session was planned in advance and a rough outline of the lesson was jotted down in a notebook. After each session, major incidents of the lesson were reflected and written down in the same notebook. Each page of the notebook was dated and entries were kept centered and each line was short so that there were enough margins on both the left and right sides, which were kept for future entries. This record was reviewed a few times during the case study.

An eye-opening experience during this case study convinced me of the potential of action research to affect personal and spiritual development. In my reflective review of my notes, simply applying the two questions introduced by van Manen (1990) to my own situation led me to a surprising awareness. The first question was "What does my student mean to me?" While I was writing my answer to this question, I was exhilarated by the potential I had to help him (e.g., I could rescue him from his predicament; I might help him to become a mathematician, etc.). However, when I asked myself the second question—"What do I mean to him?"—I felt my existence shrink to almost nothing in the context of his busy social life as a teenager with many friends, and myself a mere tutor with whom he met only once a week. This experience taught me that a simple shift of focus or difference in my way of framing an issue could cause a dramatic change in my view of my role and myself. This insight came all of a sudden, within a matter of a few minutes. I was reminded of an image in the novel *Yukiguni* (Snow Country) by Yasunari Kawabata, a Nobel Laureate in literature: "After a long tunnel, I found myself in a snow country" (1945, 5, my own translation). You can imagine the striking contrast between the gloomy dim-lit interior of a steam locomotive train confined in a completely dark tunnel and the suddenly stretched-out dazzling whiteness of the scenery. The contrast with my former way of thinking, and the unexpected view, flabbergasted me. That experience was not simply cognitive one, but my entire Chigen seemed to be shaken by the realization that action research experience can open up magnificent awakening moment over and over again.

Fatherhood

During one winter break I was dismayed to sense that the quality of the time I spent with my family had not changed significantly during the Christmas vacation, in spite of the relief I experienced from the pressure of a new job. The roots of this feeling go deep in my personal life. Traditionally in Japan childcare has been almost entirely in women's hands, while men have dedicated themselves to their occupations. I have very little memory of childhood activities with my own father. Even after learning about new roles as a father when I joined the Church of Jesus Christ of Latter-day Saints, and observing many good examples of fatherhood, I had not been able to make significant changes between my own life and my father's. These conditions motivated me to look for a breakthrough in my fatherhood by engaging in action research.

Although I was not sure what kind of improvement could be expected from such an action research, previous experience convinced me that it would certainly have an impact in my personal life. Without organizing very much at first, but expecting organization to grow out of keeping a log, I started carrying my log with me whenever it would be possible to jot down my observations of and thoughts about my family, including myself.

Action research in practice is a messy, nonlinear, dynamic, and unpredictable process. At the beginning I did not know where and how I should keep a log. On a few days I could not find time to write. At one time I found myself sitting halfway down the stairs to observe and write about my daughter, who was at the dining table on the first floor playing by herself with some kind of card. Another time I sat on the floor in the corner opposite our family computer with which my son was deeply involved. Sometimes I lay on my bed and reviewed and reflected on the accounts in the log.

Gradually I began to feel that describing what the children were doing was no longer very interesting, and I looked for further ideas. Trying to write a story about each child's life from his or her perspective turned out to be more meaningful at that point. One example is the following story I wrote from my daughter's viewpoint. She loves animals, and I tried to imagine what she might feel about recent events in her life.

> Yesterday, Josh [her older brother], Daddy and I got to give Teddy [her dog] a bath. I'm so excited, because I haven't gotten to touch Teddy for more than a week, since my skin reacts really badly to poison ivy, and Teddy is always running through places and picking up poison ivy. But since he's getting a bath today, I'll get to bring him into the house and play with him all day!

Writing these stories made me think deeply about our relationship and almost made me cry at times. I wondered how many times these important events of my children's lives went by without my noticing them. I realized that time spent together, including daily prayer as a family, does not necessarily guarantee genuine understanding, even of my own children. My usual attitude blocks some important information about my children from coming to my attention. This realization, which I had not had during fifteen years' experience with my children, came gradually throughout the whole experimental process of action research on my personal life.

From the new understanding born of writing these stories, I examined myself in reflection. I found that I was preoccupied with the idea that I must be engaged in some meaningful enterprise all the time, a sense which may have come from my diligent parents or from Japanese tradition. I noticed that being together in the same room—which seemed to free me from the guilt feelings of being a completely indifferent father—did not mean that we shared lived experiences so that we could learn about each other more deeply. When I realized that I had to do more than just be physically present, my attitude gradually began to change. I have become less frustrated by my children's responses to my requests or expectations. I do not ask unduly demanding tasks from the children as often as I did before, and my children have begun to listen to me more.

One of the results of this case study is that I have felt the need to change the nature of the attention I give my children. I decided to be completely attentive, at least for certain periods of time. My attention level has gone up and down over the period of one and a half years of this study. Then, while my wife took our daughter to Japan for schooling for a month during the early summer of the following year, I had an opportunity to care for our teenage son by myself, and I decided to use this time to give him additional attention. I faced the situation with mixed feelings of expectation and anxiety. My son is a typical "mother's child" who still "sticks" to his mother. Communication between him and me has not usually lasted long without my wife's presence. I decided to create a space in my life in which nothing could distract me from giving him my undivided attention.

After returning from summer school and finishing his homework, my son almost never failed to come to his favorite spot at home—the computer. Without drawing his attention to my purpose, I would sit or lie on the couch near the computer and give him my complete attention. The result was that our TV was not turned on for the month. I learned a great deal about why writing e-mail to his friends engages my son so much, and about his experiences in summer school, his friends, and his desires. We shared much laughter. I felt that our relationship improved. After this experience, I have this message for fathers: even though you are on the same couch or in the same room, if your mind and heart are on a TV program or something other than your child, you will not truly become acquainted with your child.

Action research about my fatherhood taught me how to shift my perspective from self-centered interpretation of others' experiences toward interpretation from their viewpoints. My experiences showed me that it is not easy to change perspective, and that change such as this requires continuous effort.

In this episode there are a few salient points to comment. First, no one asked me to undertake this case study. It was my recurring sense of inadequacy that importuned me to start this action research. Thus, I had perfect control over the course of this project; in other words, I had genuine ownership. I did not have a grand plan for this enterprise. At the beginning, I was quite uncertain about what to do, in what sequence I would do things, and so forth except for the bottom-line: keeping record of my observation. Although the two major turning points seemed to happen by chance, they led me to well-suited awareness and activities. One was the concoction of the 'story making' technique, which opened my eyes to the importance of quality attention. The other one was the experimentation of the newly acquired attitude—'undivided attention.' The grand plan that had been developed somewhere else could not possibly tell me when the best timing to try this undertaking would be. It was a locally stationed action research that could adequately address this particular kind of issue. My wife's absence could have been wasted and I could have spent an awkward summer with my son, if that action research project had not been set off before. The summer that I shared with my son never happened the way it did if there had not been the preliminary study of action research that brought up to me the issue of quality attention.

We are the ones who decide whether or not we should employ action research in our personal or professional development. We have to carefully ask ourselves whether or not such and such issue is personally valuable enough to do action research on it, because it is not without "opportunity cost." Many hours of observation, record keeping, reflection, and action were the price that allowed me to realize my near-sightedness and cultural blindness, which had rarely come to my notice because they were fully embedded in my routine. "Is it truly valuable to continue this action research enterprise to lift my fatherhood further?" Such is the query that I must ask myself repeatedly; this is a spiritual labor indeed.

Family game

The next case study is personally embarrassing, but it is a useful illustration of the impact action research can have on our views of ourselves even through trivial projects that originate from playfulness. When we engage in it wholeheartedly, an action research guides us to experiences in which we learn helpful but often unexpected or even shocking truths about ourselves.

A chance rediscovery by our son of an old computer game named Tetris resulted in an exciting experience for our family during the winter's vacation in the following year. At first nobody in the family seemed to have much interest in that game, but we decided to play a few rounds of it since we did not have anything special to do on that day. We took several turns, each of us trying to beat the score of the previous players, and as we played we all became deeply interested. Our two computers were heavily used, exclusively for this game for about two weeks.

Competition was very keen, and the outcome was perhaps predictable. Our son, with extremely quick keystrokes arising from good coordination and the ability to make fast judgments, was far ahead of anyone else. My wife, who has high technical proficiency in a variety of areas including piano, mastered the basic skills of the game quickly and had the second highest scores. Our daughter followed her, and I was last. In the heat of the competition, I thought, "How can I recover my honor? Maybe action research would work." (I wonder if anyone ever had such a thought.)

So it was my selfish desire that started this action research case study. During the daytime everyone wanted to play, and since I didn't have as much practice time as I wanted, I spent time observing others' performances and keeping a log. Some nights I played after the rest of family went to bed, and recorded all my scores and my observations. One night I did this until five o'clock in the morning.

The result? In scoring, I was still at the bottom. Yet I did make a few interesting discoveries. Based on new knowledge I acquired by keeping a record and analyzing data, my coaching helped other family members improve their performances, and I came across one innovative strategy which, when I shared it with the others, almost doubled our scores.

Then I made a shocking discovery that came to me suddenly as I was reflecting upon the data and upon my game performance. I realized that my performance style was a miniature of my life. I noticed that my weakness lies in the fact that when I face an unexpected crisis, I become overly disoriented and make errors due to slower information processing and feelings of panic. As I pondered many life experiences from my past, I realized that this weakness of mine has repeatedly caused frustrations, disharmonies, and contentions in my family. I was overwhelmed that the mere study of a game placed an understanding of one of the most fundamental problems in my life right in front of my eyes.

Reflecting on these three case studies through the windows of the five principles, what can be inferred about these components? Without true ownership, I would not have made these discoveries. It was my own desires, needs, and ideas that initiated action research. I owned the methodology, procedures, data, responsibilities, and right to organize the entire study. How can anyone commit himself or herself to serious learning in the absence of these conditions that only ownership provides? I am certain that ownership is the crucial element for deep learning.

I learned of various ideals and examples that may improve my personal life, but until I developed understanding of my own situation—locality, I could not make significant changes in my life. The idea that my problem lies in quality attention would never occur to me if I had not observed and reflected on my interaction with my children and if I had not used the make-story strategy to carefully reflect the local reality. Knowledge such as this, except for through an intimate counseling process, can only be obtained through locally oriented approaches like action research. Every turning point in my case studies was dependent upon the local knowledge produced in relation to my concerns. In the first case study, with my concern—How can I effectively help my student?—in the back of my mind, I gathered pertinent information about his interest and circumstances, which served as the basis to meaningfully ask van Manen's two questions. Without that specific information, those two discerning questions should have remained sterile. In order to obtain such knowledge, I had to be more vigilant and diligent than usual in observing and reflecting on that local reality. New insights like those that I gained were very unlikely to have been obtained through the ordinary process of everyday practice, even though I do not deny that exceptionally thoughtful practitioners may gain similar insights without consciously being engaged in action research.

Our practice requires physical, emotional, and spiritual labor, in the midst of which we unexpectedly encounter our deeper reality. Such labor is the price we must pay to obtain new insight. My experiences in these case studies taught me that being engaged in practice means exposing myself to the external world. We learn of ourselves through that projected image. Learning about ourselves does not occur in a vacuum, and our practice provides the substance that meaningfully fills the space.

We do not know the goal or destination from the outset of our action research study. We learn bit by bit through a dialectical process. I observed that this dialectical process helped me learn and grow both within each case study and among these studies. Even if at the beginning of each study I was very uncertain about what to focus on and what would be expected in the study, keeping and reviewing a log helped me remain organized. While I was writing about and reflecting on any thought and question, one idea generated another, one question led to more specifications of the study procedure, and so forth, until a clear picture of the whole study process gradually emerged.

A similar dialectical process could be found in the relationships among these three case studies. The first case study opened my eyes to the potentials of its impact on my awareness of myself. The second study led me to the point where such awareness caused changes in my life. The third case study, even though it started with personal and seemingly trivial motives, made me face a fundamental problem in my life. Each time my awareness level went deeper. For this reason, a dialectical process seems to be the key element in meaningful continuous growth.

Our deeper reality is uncovered in reflection. I witnessed that all of my important findings were born in reflection, especially while I was keeping a log and reviewing it. More accurately, some ideas may have been born in very primitive form in practice, but I feel strongly that without careful reflection they would never have developed fully enough to be called important findings. As far as I have learned in these studies, reflection is the only stage where we not only gain new awareness but also can fully develop it.

Three modes of reflection are a flowerbed from which we can hope for the never-ending germination of ideas. In my case, record, review, and report are not always separate activities. Especially while I am reviewing, I am also recording, since the margins are regularly handy and a new mind-set is a prolific writer. Record, review, and report are compared to hop-step-jump; when we reflect in report-writing thinking about the audience, the quality of reflection jumps to a new height.

Facilitation of a Student's Implementation

Once we have learned the basic empowering principles of action research, we should be able to expand application far beyond the traditional fields. The next case study suggests an innovative adaptation of action research as a comprehensive learning strategy. During the fall of 2002 I received a visit from one of my language class students. He was falling behind in my class despite the hard effort he put into learning. In fact, he was doing poorly in all of the courses that he was taking during that semester, with the resulting semester GPA of 2.0.

What I tried was to mindfully invite him to apply action research to his learning process, which turned out to be an exceptionally empowering learning experience.

Eventually he improved his learning to such a degree that after one year and a few months his name was on the dean's list. Reflecting on this experience, I noticed a pattern through which action research works in a personal development. The notable point here is that we have to have a reasonable expectation for action research. Most of the time, action research cannot be a quick remedy. However, even though it may have a slow and laborious beginning, it can bring about phenomenal results in due time. The change is not like a linear upward line or an arithmetic progression; it is not as predictably constant. It rather looks like a geometric progression or an exponential curve. If not, for some cases, these visual representations may fall short of the perfect fit. Such changes might be categorized topological: the change in quality or relational nature rather than quantity.

There seem to be three major stages in a successful implementation: the latent stage of preparation, the stage of gradual development, and the stage of sudden boost.

1. **Latent Stage of Preparation**: In this stage, the participants may not feel any tangible changes yet. Curiosity and willingness to learn about action research and learning strategies in general must sustain this stage. Support and encouragement may be more important than in the other stages. In this case study, the first several weeks or the first few months until the beginning of the next semester may be categorized as this stage.

2. **Stage of Gradual Development**: This stage is characterized as "trial and error" or "experimental period." The participants try many ideas including their own, those learned from their peers, and the ideas they learn from the learning strategy literature. This experimental stage is an adjustment period that is typically mixed with failures/mistakes/waste of time and some successes. This period is also the time when they learn themselves. In this case study, the second semester was such a period. The student's GPA improved from 2.0 to 2.75.

3. **Stage of Sudden Boost**: Throughout rather chaotic and uncertain period of Stage 2, those seemingly unrelated or random ideas/activities for improvement gradually come to form a coherent and organized whole—a system of learning improvement. Then, "ah ha!" moment arrives somewhat suddenly. Thereafter, rapid improvement ensues. In this case study, at the

beginning of the fall 2003, the student has already gone through such a critical realization and become confident enough to add extra course to his fulltime load and eventually attain the semester GPA of 3.72 with his 125% workload.

More details of this case study were found in my technical report (Ariizumi, Submitted).

Professional Performance

In this section about longitudinal case study, I reflect on the action research on my professional performance (teaching) and demonstrate how our practice reality is complex and messy. Accordingly, breakthroughs in improvement are unevenly distributed over the years for which action research has been applied. This eight-year experience has a very weak beginning. Despite my ardent desire to apply action research in my professional development, the reality of practice did not always allow me to concentrate on action research especially at the beginning of a new job. Developing courses and dealing with daily tasks consumed almost my entire time, leaving little time to keep record and reflect upon it. My attention was spread thinly over hundreds of different aspects of the job, and I had few clues to prioritize my focus. Thus, the beginning was hardly different from the learning from the experience that any practitioner may naturally have.

During the breaks between semesters, however, there was more time to plan and reflect. Some minor renovations occurred periodically over such breaks. Yet, the following several years saw only sporadic breakthroughs and many ups and downs, even though I could grow accustomed to the work and could perform the same tasks more efficiently. Persistence plays a significant role in the application of action research. Very often you cannot predict the course of the action research. Unexpectedly, the last two years became more productive. My book project on Eleanor H. Jorden's (the author of our textbooks) pedagogical contributions significantly increased the weight of the research aspect of my job responsibility. My attendance to her intensive 8-week pedagogical workshop based on the Lafayette College advanced study grant during the summer of 2002 and the implementation of the ideas from the workshop in the fall of 2002 marked a paramount turning point in my teaching performance. Serious and careful scrutiny of my teaching practice through the eyes of an expert prepared me for major breakthroughs. I describe "prepared" here because any excellent idea must be implanted carefully into the reality of practice, which process can be markedly more refined and meaningful through action research. Nevertheless, the new teaching venture in the first round of the 2002-3 school year was still unpolished. During the second year, the many scattered pieces information I had accumulated over the years came to fit together like a jigsaw puzzle. The action research cycle of Preparation, Acting/Fact Finding, and Reflection worked more coherently at both micro and macro levels in the curriculum.

For example, through streamlining the curriculum I could pay more attention to essential elements of the course suggested by the expert. I started writing in the log daily after each class and placed the log in the same file with the lesson plans bound together in a chronological order. Thus, when the semester was over I could go over the data of the entire semester at one sitting, mark the major issues, write in remarks and solutions, and list important points as the checklist to implement in the next semester. This review/plan process could be as little as 30-60 minutes. The checklist was posted on the wall so that I could review it repeatedly during the following semester.

Action research was no longer a stranger in this pedagogical undertaking; it became an integrative part of the curriculum. The results were phenomenal. Students were energized and happy, and I felt my job was largely fulfilling class after class during the entire fall semester of 2003. The students' evaluation for instructor's contribution to the course (4.9 out of 5.0 during this semester while my usual score fluctuated between 3.5 and 4.2 for the previous 7 years) also supported this memorable improvement.

The last two case studies exemplified the pattern of action research development. At the beginning, there is a certain degree of uncertainty and improvement may be modest or gradual. However, once seemingly unrelated pieces of information that action research is producing become connected one after another in a meaningful manner, it has the potential to generate a dynamite effect on improvement. The second point to remark is that the course of action research is unpredictable. An event sequence such as a book project—grant opportunity—workshop—restructuring the course—phenomenal results in my case was highly accidental. We must utilize the opportunities that are locally available. Each local situation is intensely different the next. Yet each locality is resourceful without exhaustion if and only if we learn how to tap it, for which action research can most congruously serves.

Questions & Activities for Better Understanding

The following questions and suggestions are intended to stimulate further thinking. It may not be productive to follow them in a rigid manner. The readers are encouraged to modify questions/suggestions or create new questions/suggestions so that they can engage in truly meaningful thinking and learning.

1. Can action research serve as a quick remedy? Why? It is, however, not appropriate to be preoccupied with any time-frame issue. If the time is ripe, a single action research cycle may yield a drastic change. Then, how can we decide the appropriate timing to employ action research in our practice?

2. Proactive Fact-finding Strategy A
Sometimes utilizing a conceptual devise (e.g., 'make-story' technique) makes a fact-finding process deeper and more productive. Identify one of the major issues that you would like to improve on. Describe the issue as many details as possible without interpreting or explaining the reasons. If it is possible, audio-record your oral description. You can decide an appropriate time frame for this activity (3-10 minutes might be enough). Transcribe the recording and add or edit if it is necessary. Pretend to be an expert in that field of training and interpret your description by providing reasons behind each described phenomenon. Don't hesitate to include wild guesses. You are the only audience; you do not mislead any one by this. Audio-record, transcribe, and add/edit your interpretation within an appropriate time frame. Based on the results of this second step, continue the exercise by giving some technical advice to improve the situation. Repeat the same procedure to get an edited writing. Now, you have a quite extensive basis for research. Using this, you may create many research questions that verify or falsify the points.

3. Proactive Fact-finding Strategy B
Carry out the same approach as a pair or a team. It is not necessary to include any sort of expert in this activity. Whoever willing to participate in this experience should be fitting for this collaboration. The advantage of collaboration is that triangulation and validity-check are naturally embedded in its process. This endeavor can be fun as well as productive in terms of diversity through the ideas that you generate.

4. In what areas or fields of activity can you meaningfully apply action research? Consider the following: the role in your work, the relationship with the key people in your life, the productivity and efficiency of your task per-

formance, your skills to organize activities and other things, your communication skills, and your spiritual strength.

5. Knowing the three stages of action research development, what attitude should you acquire so that you can steadily move on through the procedure?

Bibliography

Adler, S. A. 1993. Teacher education: Research as reflective practice. *Teaching and Teacher Education*, 2, 159-167.
Altrichter, H., Posch, P., & Somekh, B. 1993. *Teachers investigate their work: An introduction to the methods of action research*. London: Routledge.
Altrichter, H., Kemmis, S., McTaggart, R., & Zuber-Skerritt, O. 1991. Defining, confining or refining action research? In *Action research for change and development*, edited by O. Zuber-Skerritt, 3-9. Brookfield: Avebuy.
Anderson, G. 1994. A proactive model for training needs analysis. *Journal of European Industrial Training*, 18(3), 23-28.
Argyris, C., & Schön, D. 1991. Participatory action research and action science compared. In *Participatory action research*, edited by W. F. Whyte, New York: Sage.
Argyris, C., & Schön, D. 1989. Participatory action research and action science compared. *American Behavioral Scientist*, 32, 612-623.
Argyris, C., Putnam, R., & Smith, D. M. 1985. *Action science*. San Francisco:

Jossey-Bass.

Ariizumi, Y. Submitted. Action research as another literacy skill to improve academic performance: A case study of empowered learning. Submitted to ERIC(Educational Resources Information Center).

Avery, C. S. 1990. Learning to research/Researching to learn. In *Opening the door to classroom research*, Edited by M.W. Olson, 32-40. Newark, DE: International Reading Association.

Baillie, A. 1996. The construction of clients' experience of psychotherapy through narrative, practical action and the multiple streams of consciousness. *Human Relations*, 49, 295-311.

Bennett, C. K. 1994. Promoting teacher reflection through action research: What do teachers think? *Journal of Staff Development*, 15(1), 34-38.

Biott, C. 1983. The foundations of classroom action-research in initial teacher training. *Journal of Education for Teaching*, 9(2), 152-160.

Bolster, A. S. 1983. Toward a more effective model of research on teaching. *Harvard Educational Review*, 53(3), 294-308.

Brooks-Carhcart, K. 1996. *Reflection on action research: Todays, tomorrows & yesterdays in my backyard* [online]. Ontario, Canada: Queen's University, 1998 [available 27 January 2005] http://educ.queensu.ca/projects/action-research/karen.htm.

Brown, J. S., Collins, A., & Duguid, P. 1989. Situated cognition and the culture of learning. *Educational Research*, 18, 32-42.

Burnaford, G., Beane, J., & Brodhagen, B. 1994. Teacher action research: Inside and integrative curriculum. *Middle School Journal*, 26(2), 3-13.

Calderhead, J. 1989. Reflective teaching and teacher education. *Teaching and teacher education*, 5(1), 43-51.

Calhoun, E. F. 1993. Action research: Three approaches. *Educational Leadership*, 51(2), 62-65.

Carr, W. ed. 1989. *Quality in teaching: Arguments for reflective professions*. London: Falmer.

Carr, W. 1980. The gap between theory and practice. *Journal of Further and Higher Education*, 20(2), 177-186.

Carson, T. 1990. What kind of knowing is critical action research? *Theory Into Practice*, 29(3), 167-173.

Cassidy, T. 1986. Initiating and encouraging action research in comprehensive schools. In *Action research in classrooms and schools* Edited by D. Hustler, A. Cassidy, & E. C. Cuff, 133-142. London: Allen & Unwin.

Chisholm, R. F., & Elden, M. 1993. Features of emerging action research. *Human Relations*, 46(2), 275-297.

Cochran-Smith, M., & Lytle, S. 1993. *Inside/Outside: Teacher research and knowledge*. New York: Teachers College Press.

Connolly, M., & Ennew, J. 1996. Introduction: Children out of place. *Childhood: Global journal of child research*, 3(2), 131-145

Corey, S. 1953. *Action research to improve school practices*. New York: Teachers College.

Cunningham, J. B. *1993*. Action research and organizational development. Westport, Connecticut: Prager.
Cumming, A. 1994. Alternatives in TESOL research: Descriptive, interpretive, and ideological orientations. *TESOL Quarterly*, 28(4), 673-703.
Dadds, M. 1993. Thinking and being in teacher action research. In *Reconstructing teacher education*. Edited by J. Elliott, 229-242. London: Falmer.
Davidoff, S., ed. 1993. Emancipatory education and action research (Action Research Series No. 1). Pretoria, South Africa: HDRS Publishers.
Davies, R. 1993. Chronicles: Doing action research: The stories of three teachers. In *Reconstructing teacher education*. Edited by J.Elliott, 145-153. London: Falmer.
Davis, N. T. 1996. Looking in the mirror: Teacher's use of autobiography and action research to improve practice. *Research in Science Education*, 26(1), 23-32.
Day, C. 1993. Reflection: A necessary but not sufficient condition for professional development. *British Educational Research Journal*, 19(1), 83-93.
Denton, J. J., & Peters, W. H. 1998. Development of reflective thinking skills about pedagogy during a fifteen month intern program. In *Images of reflection in teacher education*, edited by H. C. Waxman, H. J. Freiberg, J. C. Vaughan, & M. Weil, 40-41. Reston, VA: Association of Teacher *Educators*.
Denzin, N. K., & Lincoln, Y. S. 1994. *Handbook of qualitative research*. London: Sage.
Ebbutt, D. 1985. Educational action research: Some general concerns and specific quibbles. In *Issues in educational research: Qualitative methods*, edited by R. G. Burgress, 152-174. East Sussex, UK: Falmer.
Ecclestone, K. 1996. The reflective practitioner: Mantra or a model or emancipation. *Studies in the Education of Adults*, 28(2), 146-161.
Eisner, E. W. 1993. The emergence of new paradigms for educational research. *Art Education*, 46(6), 50-55.
Elden, M., & Chisholm, R. F. 1993. Emerging varieties of action research: Introduction to the special issue. *Human Relations*, 46, 121-142.
Elliott, J. 1993. Academics and action-research: The training workshop as an exercise in ideological deconstruction. In *Reconstructing teacher education*, J. Elliott, 176-192. London: Falmer.
Elliott, J. 1991b. Changing contexts for educational evaluation: The challenge for methodology. *Studies in Educational Evaluation*, 17(2-3), 215-238.
Elliott, J. 1991a. *Action research for educational change*. Philadelphia: Open University Press.
Elliott, J. 1989. Teacher evaluation and teaching as a moral science. In *Perspectives on teacher professional development*, edited by M. L. Holly, & C. S. Mcloughlin, 239-258. London: Falmer.
Elliott, J. 1989. *Academic and action-research: The training workshop as an exercise in ideological deconstruction*. Paper presented at the meeting of American Educational Research Association, San Francisco, CA.

Elliott, J. 1987. Educational theory, practical philosophy and action research. *British Journal of Educational Studies*, 35(2), 149-169.

Errington, E. P. 1993. Teachers as researchers: Pursing qualitative enquiry in drama classrooms. *Youth Theatre Journal*, 7(4), 31-36.

Evans, K. S. 1995. Teacher reflection as a cure for tunnel vision. *Language Arts*, 72, 266-271.

Fals-Borda, L, & Rahman, M. A., eds. 1991. *Action and knowledge: Breaking the monopoly with participatory action research*. New York: Apex Press.

Feinman, L. 1991. Action research in retrospect: Does she or doesn't she? *Hands On*, 39, 60-64.

Feldman, A., & Atkin, J. M. 1995. Embedding action research in professional practice. In *Educational action research: Becoming practically critical*, edited by S. E. Noffke, & R. B. Stevenson, 127-137. New York: Teacher College Press.

Feldman, A. 1994. Erzberger's dilemma: Validity in action research and science teacher's need to know. *Science Education*, 78(1), 83-101.

Fellows, K, & Zimpher, N. L. 1988. Reflectivity and the instructional process: A definitional comparison between theory and practice. In *Images of reflection in teacher education*, edited by H. C. Waxman, H. J. Freiberg, J. C. Vaughan, & M. Weil, 18-19. Reston, VA: Association of Teacher Educators.

Fisher, C. W., & Berliner, D. C. 1979. Critical inquiry in research on classroom teaching and learning. *Journal of Teacher Education*, 30(6), 42-48.

Fleischer, C. 1994. Researching teacher-research: A practitioner's retrospective. *English Education*, 26(2), 86-124.

Flores, E., & Granger, S. 1995. The role of the collaborator in action research. In *Educational action research: Becoming practically critical*, edited by S. E. Noffke, & Stevenson, R. B., 165-179. New York: Teachers College Press.

Foshay, A. W. 1994. Action research: An early history in the United States. *Journal of Curriculum and Supervision*, 9(4), 317-325.

Friere, P. 1972. *Pedagogy of the oppressed*. Harmonsworth: Penguin.

Gebhard, J. G. (1989, March). The teacher as investigator of classroom processes: Procedures and benefits. Paper presented at the meeting of the Teachers of English to Speakers of Other Languages, San Antonio, TX.

George, J. W. 1996. Action research for quality development in rural education in Scotland. *Journal of Research in Rural Education*, 12(2), 76-82.

Gianotti, M. A. 1994. Moving between two worlds: Talk during writing workshop. In *Changing schools from within*, edited by G. Wells, 37-59. Portsmouth, NH: Heinemann.

Glaser, B. G. 1978. *Theoretical sensitivity*. Millvalley, CA: The Sociology Press.

Glesne, C. E. 1991. Yet another role? The teacher as researcher. *Action in Teacher Education*, 13(1), 7-13.

Goodlad, J. I. 1976. *Facing the future*. New York: McGraw-Hil

Goswani, D., & Stillman, P. R., eds. 1987. *Reclaiming the classroom: Teacher research as an agency for change.* Upper Montclair, NJ: Boynton Cook.

Greenwood, D. J. 1993. Participatory action research as a process and as a goal. *Human Relations*, 46(2), 175-192.

Griffiths, M., & Davies, C. 1993. Learning to learn: Action research from an equal opportunities perspective in a junior school. *British Educational Research Journal*, 19(1), 43-58.

Grimmett, P. P. 1996. The struggles of teacher research in a context of education reform: Implications for instructional supervision. *Journal of Curriculum and Supervision*, 12(1), 37-65

Gustavsen, B. 1993. Action research and the generation of knowledge. *Human Relations*, 46, 1361-1365.

Habermas, J. 1972. Knowledge and human interests. Translated by J. Shapiro. Boston: Beacon Press.

Hamilton, M. L. 1995. Relevant readings in action research. *Action in Teacher Education*, 16(4), 79-81.

Hargreaves, A. 1997. Rethinking educational change: Going deeper and wider in the quest for success. In, *Rethinking educational change with heart and mind*, edited by A. Hargreaves, 1-26. Alexandria, VA: Association for Supervision and Curriculum Development.

Heidegger, M. 1962. *Being and time* [translated by John Macquarrie and Edward Robinson]. San Francisco: Harper.

Heller, F. A. 1993. Another look at action research. *Human Relations*, 46, 1235-1242.

Heron, J. 1981. Philosophical basis for a new paradigm. In *Human Inquiry*, edited by P. Reason, & J. Rowan, 19-35. New York: John Wiley & Sons.

Hendry, C. 1996. Understanding and creating whole organizational change through learning theory. *Human Relations*, 49, 621-641.

Herrick, M. J. 1992. Research by the teacher and for the teacher: An action research model linking schools and universities. *Action in Teacher Education*, 14(3), 47-54.

Hogan, P., & Clandinin, D. J. 1993. Living the story of received knowing: Constructing a story of connected knowing. In *Learning to teach, teaching to learn*, edited D. J. Clandinin, A. Davies, P. Hogan, & B. Kennard (Eds.) (pp. 193-199). New York: Teachers College Press.

Hollingsworth, S. 1992. Teachers as researchers: A review of the literature (Occasional paper No. 142). East Lansing, MI: Institute for Research on Teaching.

Holly, P. 1991. From action research to collaborative enquiry: The processing of an innovation. In *Action research for change and development*, edited by O. Zuber-Skerritt, 36-56. Brookfield: Avebury.

Hopkins, D. 1993. *A teacher's guide to classroom research.* Buckingham: Open University Press.

Hopkins, D. 1987. Teacher research on teacher research. In B. Somekh, Norman, B. Shannon, & G. Abbott, eds. *Action research in development*, 102-

108 (Classroom Action Research Network Bulletin, No. 8). Cambridge: Cambridge Institute of Education.

Houston, W. R. 1988. Reflecting on reflection in teacher education. In *Images of reflection in Teacher education*, edited H. C. Waxman, H. J. Freiberg, J. C. Vaughan, & M. Weil, 7-8). Reston, VA: Association of Teacher Educators.

Hustler, D., Cassidy, A., & Cuff, E. C., eds. 1986. *Action research in classrooms and schools*. London: Allen & Unwin.

Isakson, M. B., & Boody, R. M. 1993. Hard questions about teacher research. In *Teachers are researchers: Reflection and action*, edited by L. Patterson, C. M. Santa, K. G. Short, & K. Smith, 26-36. Newark: International Reading Association.

James, P. 1996. Learning to reflect: A story of empowerment. *Teaching and Teacher Education*, 12(1), 81-97.

Johnson, R. W. 1993. Where can teacher research lead? One teacher's daydream. *Educational Leadership*, 51(2), 66-68.

Johnston, S., & Proudford, C. 1994. Action research--who owns the process? *Educational Review*, 46(1), 3-14.

Joyappa, V.& Martin, D. T. 1996. Exploring alternative research epistemologies for adult education: Participatory research, feminist research and feminist participatory research. *Adult Education Quarterly*, 47(1), 1-14.

Kaplan, L. 1976. Survival talk for educators--The teacher as researcher. *Journal of Teacher Educator*, 27(1), 67-68.

Kawabata, Y. 1945. *Yukiguni*. Tokyo: Shinchosha.

Kelly, A. 1985. Action research: What is it and what can it do? In *Issues in educational research: Qualitative methods*, edited by R. G. Burgress, 129-151. London: Falmer.

Kelly, G. A. 1963. *A theory of personality*. New York: Norton.

Kember, D., & Gow, L. 1992. Action research as a form of staff development in higher education. *Higher Education*, 23(3), 297-310.

Kemmis, S. 1994. Action research. In The International Encyclopedia of Education 2nd ed., edited by T. Husen & T. N. Postlethwaite. 35-42. New York: Pergamon.

Kemmis, S., & Dichiro, G. (1987). Emerging and evolving issues of action research praxis: An Australian perspective. *Peabody Journal of Education*, 64, 101-130.

Kemmis, S. (1980, November). Action research in retrospect and prospect. Paper presented at the meeting of the Australian Association for Research in Education, Sidney.

Kincheloe, J. L. 1991. *Teachers as researchers: Qualitative inquiry as a path to empowerment*. London: Falmer.

King, J. A., & Lonnquist, M. P. 1992. *A review of writing on action research (1944-present)*. Madison, WI: Center on Organization and Restructuring of Schools.

Kosmidou, C., & Usher, R. 1991. Facilitation in action research. *Interchange*, 22(4), 24-40.

Kroath, F. 1989. How do teachers change their practical theories? *Cambridge Journal of Education*, 19(1), 59-69.

Kyle, P. W., & Hovda, R. A. 1987. Teachers as action researchers: A discussion of developmental, organizational, and policy issues. *Peabody Journal of Education*, 64(2), 80-95.

Lasky, L. R. 1978. Personalizing teaching: Action research in action. *Young Children*, 33(3), 58-64.

Lather, P. 1986. Research as praxis. *Harvard Educational Review*, 56(3), 257-277.

Ledford, G. E., & Mohrman, S. A. 1993. Looking backward and forward at action research. *Human Relations*, 46, 1349-1359.

Letiche, H. 1987. Facilitation fallacies. In *Action research in development*, edited by B. Somekh, A. Norman, B. Shannon, & G. Abbott, 86-93. (Classroom Action Research Network Bulletin, No. 8). Cambridge: Cambridge Institute of Education.

Lewin, K. 1947. Frontiers in group dynamics II. Channels of group life: Social planning and action research. *Human Relations*, 1(2), 143-153.

Lewin, K. 1946. Action research and minority problems. *Journal of Social Issues*, 2(4), 34-46.

Lewin, K., & Grabbe, P. 1945. Conduct, knowledge, and acceptance of new values. *Journal of Social Issues*, 1(3), 53-64.

Longstreet, W. S. 1982. Action research: A paradigm. *Educational Forum*, 46(2), 135-158.

Lytle, S. L., Cockran-Smith, M. 1992. Teacher research as a way of knowing. *Harvard Educational Review*, 62(4), 447-474.

MacKinnon, A., & Erickson, G. 1992. The roles of reflective practice and Foundational disciplines. In *Teachers and teaching: From classroom to reflection*, edited by T. Russell, & H. Munby, London: Falmer.

Mangham, I. L. 1993. Conspiracies of silence? Some critical comments on the action research special issue, February 1993. *Human Relations*, 46, 1243-1251.

Manicas, P. T., & Secord, P. F. 1983. Implications for psychology of the new philosophy of science. *American Psychologist*, 38, 399-413.

Marshak, R. J. 1993. Lewin meets confucius: A re-view of the OD model of change. *Journal of Applied Behavioral Science*, 29(4), 393-415.

Maruyama, G. 1992. Lewin's impact on education: Instilling cooperation and conflict management skills in school children. *Journal of Social Issues*, 48(2), 155-166.

McCutcheon, G., & Jung, B. 1990. Alternative perspectives on action research. *Theory Into Practice*, 29(3), 144-151.

McElroy, L. 1990. Becoming real: An ethic at the heart of action research. *Theory Into Practice*, 29(3), 209-213.

McFarland, K. P., & Stansell, J. C. 1993. Historical perspectives. In *Teachers are researchers: Reflection and Action*, edited by L. Patterson, C. M. Santa,

K. G. Short, & K. Smith, 12-18. Newark: International Reading Association.

McKay, J. 1992. Professional development through action research. *Journal of Staff Development*, 13(1), 18-21.

McKay, J. 1991. *Teacher as action researcher: The key to middle level reform* (Practitioner's Monograph No. 12). Irvine, CA: California League of Middle School.

McKernan, J. 1991. *Curriculum Action Research*. New York: St. Martin's Press.

McKernan, J. 1988. Teacher as researcher: Paradigm and praxis. *Contemporary Education*, 59(3), 154-158.

McKernan, J. 1988. The coutenance of curriculum action research: Traditinal, collaborative, and emancipatory-critical conceptions. *Journal of Curriculum and Supervision*, 3(3), 173-200.

McNiff, J. 1988. *Action research: Principles and practice*. London: Macmillan.

McTaggart, R., ed. 1997. *Participatory action research: International contexts and consequences*. Albany: State University of New York Press.

McTaggart, R. 1988. *Action research: A prologue to praxis*. Geelong, Victoria: Deakin University Press.

Miller, N. 1994. Participatory action research: Principles, politics, and possibilities. *New Directions for Adult and Continuing Education*, 63, 69-80.

Nash, J. D. 1987. Action research in a CPVE communications group: Why action research? In *Action research in development*, edited by B. Somekh, A. Norman, B. Shannon, & G. Abbott, 139-145 (Classroom Action Research Network Bulletin, No. 8). Cambridge: Cambridge Institute of Education.

Newby, M. J. 1997. Educational action research: The death of meaning? or, The practitioner's response to utopian discourse. *Educational Research*, 39(1), 77-86.

Nixon, J. 1987. The teacher as researcher: Contradictions and continuities. *Peabody Journal of Education*, 64(2), 20-32.

Noffke, S. E. 1995. Action research and democratic schooling. In *Educational action research: Becoming practically critical*, edited by S. E. Noffke, & Stevenson, R. B., 1-10. New York: Teachers College Press.

Noffke, S. E. 1994. Action research: Towards the next generation. *Action Research*, 2(1), 9-21.

Noffke, S. E. (1990). *Action research: A multidimensional analysis*. Doctoral dissertation, University of Wisconsin-Madison.

Nyden, P., & Wiewel, W. 1992. Collaborative research: Harnessing the tensions between researcher and practitioner. *American Sociologist*, 23(4), 43-55.

Oberg, A. 1990. Methods and meanings in action research: The action research journal. *Theory Into Practice*, 29(3), 214-221.

Oberg, A., & McCutcheon, G. 1987. Teachers' experience doing action research. *Peabody Journal of Education*, 64(2), 116-127.

Oja, S. N., & Smulyan, L. 1989. *Collaborative action research: A developmental approach*. London: Falmer.

Oja, S. N., & Ham, M. C. 1984. A cognitive-developmental approach to collaborative action research with teachers. *Teachers College Record*, 86(1), 171-192.

Olsen, M. W. 1990. The teacher as researcher: A historical perspective. In *Opening the door to classroom research*, edited by M. W. Olsen, Newark Del.: International Reading Association.

Pace, L. A. 1989. Participatory action research: A view from Xerox. *American Behavioral Scientist*, 32, 552-565.

Pajares, M. F. 1992. Teachers' beliefs and educational research: Cleaning up a messy construct. *Review of Educational Research*, 62(3), 307-332.

Pareek, U. 1990. Culture-relevant and culture-modifying action research for development: Part of a symposium: Psychology for the third world. *Journal of Social Issues*, 46(3), 119-131.

Patterson, L., & Stansell, J. C. (1987). Teachers and researchers: A new matualism. *Language Arts*, 64(7), 717-721.

Peake, L. 1992. Devising motor programs for children with physical disabilities. In *Teacher research and special education needs*, edited by G. Vulliamy & R. Webb, London: David Fulton.

Pedretti, E., & Hodson, D. 1995. From rhetoric to action: Implementing STS education through action research. *Journal of Research in Science Teaching*, 32, 463-485.

Piaget, J. 1977. The role of action in the development of thinking. In *Knowledge and development I. Advances in research and theory*, edited by W. F. Overton & J. M. Gallagher, New York: Plenum Press.

Polanyi, M. 1969. *Knowing and being*. London: Routledge and Kegan Paul.

Polanyi, M. 1958. *Personal knowledge: Towards a post-critical philosophy*. Chicago: The University of Chicago Press.

Prendergast, M. 1996. *Seven stages in my first action research project* [online]. Ontario, Canada, Queen's University, Action Research at Queen's University, 1998 [Available 27 January 2005] from Wold Wide Web: (http://educ.queensu.ca/projects/action_research/michael.htm)

Quigley, B. A. 1995. Action research for professional development and policy formation in literacy education. *PAACE Journal of Lifelong Learning*, 4, 61-69.

Reason, P. 1993. Sitting between appreciation and disappointment: A critique of the special edition of Human Relations on action research. *Human Relations*, 46, 1253-1270.

Richardson, V. 1990. The evolution of reflective teaching and teacher education. In *Encouraging reflective practice in education*, edited by R.T. Clift, W. R. Houston, & M. C. Pugach, 3-19. New York: Teachers College Press.

Rist, R. 1982. Foward. In *Qualitative research for education: An introduction to theory and methods*, edited by R. C. Bogdan & S. K. Biklen, Boston: Allyn and Bacon Inc.

Roberts, J. R. 1993. Evaluating the impacts of teacher research. *System*, 21(1), 1-19.

Ross, D. D. 1988. Reflective teaching: Meaning and implications for pre-service teacher educators. In *Images of reflection in Teacher education*, edited by H. C. Waxman, H. J. Freiberg, J. C. Vaughan, & M. Weil, 25-26. Reston, VA: Association of Teacher Educators.

Ross, D. D. 1984. A practical model for conducting action research in public school settings. *Contemporary Education*, 55(2), 113-117.

Rudduck, J., & Hopkins, D., eds. 1985. *Research as a basis forteaching: Readings from the work of Lawrence Stenhouse*. London: Heinemann.

Sands, D., & Drake, S. 1996. Exploring a process for delivering and interdisciplinary pre-service elementary education curriculum: Teacher educators practice what they preach. *Action in Teacher Education*, 18(3), 68-79.

Sardo-Brown, D. 1992. Elementary teachers' perceptions of action research. *Action in Teacher Education*, 14(2), 55-59.

Secord, P. 1984. Determinism, free will, and self-intervention: A psychological perspective. *New Ideas in Psychology*, 2, 25-33.

Shalaway, L. 1990. Tap into teacher research. *Instructor*, 100(1), 34-38.

Sharples, D. (1983, March). An overview of school based action research. Paper presented at Action Research in Classrooms and Schools Conference. Manchester Polytechnic.

Sockett, H. (1989, March). The challenge to action-research. Paper presented at the meeting of the American Educational Research Association, San Francisco.

SooHoo, S. (1989, March). Teacher researcher: Emergent change agent. Paper presented at the meeting of the American Educational Research Association, San Francisco.

Sparks-Langer, G. M. 1993. In the eye of the beholder: Cognitive, critical, and narrative approaches to teacher reflection. In *Reconstruting teacher education*, edited by J. Elliott, 147-160. London: Falmer.

Stenhouse, L. 1983. The relevance of practice to theory. *Theory into Practice*, 22(3), 211-215.

Stenhouse, L. 1981. What counts as research? *British Journal of Educational Studies*, 29, 103-114.

Stenhouse, L. 1975. *An introduction to curriculum research and development*. London: Heinemann.

Stevenson, R. B., Noffke, S. E., Flores, E., & Granger, S. 1995. Teaching action research: A case study. In *Educational action research: Becoming practically critical*, edited by S. E. Noffke, & Stevenson, R. B., 60-73. New York: Teachers College Press.

Stevenson, R. B. 1995. Action research and supportive school contexts. In *Educational action research: Becoming practically critical*, edited by S. E. Noffke, & Stevenson, R. B., 197-209. New York: Teachers College Press.

Strickland, D. S. 1988. The teacher as researcher: Toward the extended professional. *Language Arts*, 65(8), 754-764.

Suchman, L. A. 1987. *Plans and situated actions. The problem of human-machine communication*. Cambridge: Cambridge University Press.

Susman, G. I., & Evered, R. D. 1978. An assessment of the scientific merits of action research. *Administrative Science Quarterly*, 23, 582-603.

Tinto, P. P., Shelly, B. A., & ZaN. J. 1994. Classroom research and classroom practice: Blurring the boundaries. *Mathematicis Teacher*, 87(8), 644-648.

Valli, L. 1990. Moral approaches to reflective practice. In *Encouraging reflective practice in education*, edited by R. T. Clift, W. R. Houston, & M. C. Pugach, 39-56. New York: Teachers College Press.

Valli, L., & Taylor, N. E. 1988. Reflective teacher education: Preferred characteristics. In *Images of reflection in Teacher education*, edited by H. C. Waxman, H. J. Freiberg, J. C. Vaughan, & M. Weil, 20-21. Reston, VA: Association of Teacher Educators.

van Manen, M. 1991a. Reflectivity and the pedagogical moment: The normativity of pedagogical thinking and acting. *Journal of Curriculum Studies*, 23(6), 507-536.

van Manen, M. 1991b. *The tact of teaching: The meaning of pedagogical thoughtfulness.* Albany: State University of New York Press.

van Manen, M. 1990. *Researching lived experience: Human science for an action sensitive pedagogy.* New York: State University of New York Press.

van Manen, M. 1986. *The tone of teaching.* Portsmouth, NH: Heinemann.

Vulliamy, G., & Webb, R., eds. 1992. *Teacher research and special educational needs.* London: David Fulton.

Wallace, M. 1987. A historical review of action research: Some implications for the education of teachers in their managerial role. *Journal of Education for Teaching*, 13(2), 97-115.

Watkins, K. E., & Brooks, A. 1994. A framework for using action technologies. *New Directions for Adult and Continuing Education*, 63, 99-111.

Wells, G. 1994. Introduction: Teacher research and educational change. In *Changing schools from within*, edited by G. Wells, 1-35. Portsmouth, NH: Heinemann.

Whiston, S. C. 1996. Accountability through action research: Research methods for practitioners. *Journal of Counseling and Development*, 74(6), 616-623.

Whitehead, J. (1994, April). Creating a living educational theory from an analysis of my own educational practice: How do you create and test the validity of your living educational theory? Paper presented at the annual meeting of the American Educational Research Association, New Orleans, LA.

Whyte, W. F. 1989. Action research for twenty-first century: introduction. *American Behavioral Scientist*, 32, 502-512.

Whyte, W. F. 1989. Advancing scientific knowledge through action research. *Sociological Forum*, 4(3), 367-385.

Wilson, C., ed. 1991. A vision of a preferred curriculum for the 21st century: Action research in school administration. Paper presented at the annual meeting of the Association for Supervision and Curriculum Development, San Francisco, CA.

Winter, R. 1989. *Learning from experience: Principles and practice in action-research.* London: Falmer.

Winter, R. 1987. *Action-research and the nature of social inquiry: Professional innovation and educational work.* Brookfield, VA: Avebury.

Yeatman, A. 1996. The roles of scientific and non-scientific types of knowledge in the improvement of practice. *Australian Journa of Education,* 40(3), 284-301.

Yinger, R. J. 1991. Thinking-in-action: Lessons from the field. In K. M. Borman, P. Swami, & L. P. Wagstaff (Eds.), Contemporary issues in U. S. education (pp. 105-127). Norwood, NJ: Ablex

Zeichner, K. M., & Liston, D. P. 1987. Teaching student teachers to reflect. *Harvard Educational Review,* 57(1), 23-48.

Zeichner, K. M. 1982. Reflective teaching and field-based experience in teacher education. *Interchange,* 12(4), 1-22.

Zinsser, W. K. 1988. *Writing to learn.* New York: Harper & Row.

Zuber-Skerritt, O. 1993. Improving learning and teaching through action learning and action research. *Higher Education Research and Development,* 12(1), 45-58.

Zuber-Skerritt, O. 1992b. *Professional development in higher education: A Theoretical framework for action research.* London: Kogan Page.

Zuber-Skerritt, O. 1992a. *Action research in higher education—Examples and reflections.* London: Kogan Page.

Zuber-Skerritt, O. 1991. Action research as a model of professional development. In *Action research for change and development,* edited by O. Zuber-Skerritt, 112-135. Brookfield, VA: Avebury.

Index

A

Ability, 20, 29, 57, 72, 92
Abstract, 2, 27, 43
Academic, 23, 34, 36
Access, 29, 73
Accept, 19, 35, 75, 77
Accomplish, 7, 39, 44, 62
Account, 7-8, 13, 16, 19-20, 22, 24, 37, 52, 59, 67, 76, 89
Accurate, 5, 8, 16, 29, 42, 74, 76, 94
Achieve, 2, 40, 68, 72
Acquire, 23, 36-7, 39, 57, 74, 78, 91-2, 99

Advance, 17, 54, 57, 62, 72-4, 88, 96
Advantage, 22, 28, 37, 47, 54-6, 79, 98
Advise, 51, 82, 98
Affect, 16, 17-21, 25, 35, 39, 41, 51-2, 57, 65, 88
Aftermath, 76
Agency, 14, 19, 20, 44, 46-48, 56-8, 62, 74, 78
Agenda, 14, 17-8
Aggressive, 55
Agree, 72
Aim, 17, 19, 24, 27, 38, 52, 64, 74, 74

Alter, 2, 4-5, 20, 41, 63-5, 69
Analysis, 2, 6, 9, 10, 30, 40, 45, 47, 60, 92
Anxiety, 39, 41, 78, 90
Apply, 1-7, 15, 25-8, 30, 40, 43, 45, 55, 59, 63-5, 68, 75, 79, 85, 88, 94-6, 98
Armchair, 39
Arrow, 65, 67, 69
Articulate, 8, 27-9, 42-3, 54-7, 60, 76-8, 80-1
Asia, 39, 64
Assign, 76
Attract, 3
Automatic, 16, 29, 57
Aware, 18, 23, 28-9, 36, 48, 57-8, 62, 73, 76-9, 81, 83, 87-8, 91, 94
Awkward, 91

B
Being, 3, 7, 10, 19, 39-48, 53, 57, 63, 93
Belong, 10, 16
Black box, 9
Blind, 25, 46, 91
Boundary, 2-4, 71
Bridge, 2-3, 33, 55, 78
Built-in, 64, 73
Butterfly, 25
Bystander, 34, 37

C
Capacity, 46, 80
Car, 16, 26
Career, 59
Casual, 3, 72, 75, 79, 86
Chart, 37-8
Complement, 8, 23-4, 40, 47, 63-4, 67, 81
Confucius, 53, 81

Connection, 2, 34, 37, 41-2, 55, 57, 72, 97
Converge, 74-5
Crook, 54

D
Dean's list, 95
Delineate, 47, 64, 86
Destination, 16, 37, 62, 93
Diagnose, 27, 46
Diverse, 35, 56, 74-5, 98
Divine, 49, 53
Dog, 10, 89
Dot, 26
Drive, 16, 28
Dynamic, 36-7, 82, 89

E
Emotion, 7, 10, 16, 21, 35, 39, 41-2, 53, 78, 93
Empower, 2, 29, 74, 85, 94-5
Enigma, 78
Equilibrium, 79
Espouse, 53-5
Ethic, 20, 52, 65, 68, 79
Evolve, 85-6

F
Facilitate, 14-22, 34-5, 46-7, 54, 64, 70, 73, 82, 85, 94
Faculty, 20, 39-41, 56-7, 67, 72, 78-82
Father, 10, 25, 85, 89-91
Feedback, 59, 81
Fighter, 9

G
Game, 39, 85, 92-3
Gem, 78

Guide, 1, 5, 24, 38, 41-2, 45, 48, 52-4, 72, 81, 92

H
Hammer, 28

J
Japan, 4, 9, 14, 39, 46, 53, 68, 81, 69-90
Journal, 80
Judgment, 8-9, 17, 20, 41, 43, 47, 54, 75-6, 79, 82, 92
Junction, 41, 74

L
Linear, 35-7, 62, 73, 89, 95
Literature, 61, 81, 84, 88, 95
Log, 40, 80, 84, 86, 89, 92, 94, 97

M
Manifest, 35, 50, 82
Metacognition, 39-40
Moral, 15, 19-20, 22, 49, 52, 54, 59, 79
Mound, 26, 64

N
Navigate, 37, 62
Novel, 55, 88

O
Opportunity, 7, 11, 14, 17-8, 21, 74, 90-1, 97
Oppress, 43
Option, 4, 9, 11, 41

P

Pacific islanders, 37
Panacea, 7
Participate, 34, 56, 95, 98
Passenger, 16
Pearl, 78
Pool, 75
Predicament, 4, 88

R
Random, 95
Refine, 6-7, 10, 26, 29, 37, 44, 47-51, 56, 64, 72, 74, 79-82, 87, 97
Relevant, 1, 4, 30, 36, 45, 54-7, 62, 73-7, 83-4
Rigor, 73-7, 83
Ripple, 25
Route, 16, 72

S
Sense, 17, 27, 41-2, 51, 59, 68, 79, 89, 90-1
Space, 18, 34, 55, 57, 69, 78, 86, 90, 93
Statistics, 43, 49, 51, 76
Subsidiary, 24, 27-8, 34, 56, 58, 73, 78-9
Superficial, 5, 16, 19, 47
Supplement, 72, 74
Sword, 9

T
Tacit, 8, 10, 27-29, 35, 42, 54-6, 60, 64, 80
Trukese, 37-8
Trustworthy, 43, 45, 49, 51-2, 59, 74
Tunnel, 88

U

Unconscious, 44
Underestimate, 25

V
Valid, 6-8, 24-5, 39, 44-5, 52, 54, 74-6, 83, 98

W
Wake, 10, 88

Z
Zen, 67-8

About the Author

Yoshihiko Ariizumi (PhD, Brigham Young University) is an assistant professor of Japanese Studies at Lafayette College. He is a third generation educator in his Japanese family. His research interest covers instructional psychology & technology, educational measurement, andragogy, linguistics, undergraduate research, and intercultural communication. His recent publication includes "Integrating Technology into the Curriculum Using Adaptive and Dynamic Features" and "More Tactful Way of Teaching Japanese Based on the Andragogical Premises."

www.ingramcontent.com/pod-product-compliance
Lightning Source LLC
Chambersburg PA
CBHW021130300426
44113CB00006B/368